Life Regained™

The Real Solution to Managing Menopause and Andropause

Gino Tutera, MD, FACOG

SottoPelle Marketing Group®

For further information, please contact:
carolann@sottopelletherapy.com

Printed in Canada

Life Regained: The Real Solution to Managing Menopause and Andropause
Dr. Gino Tutera

1. Title 2. Author 3. Health

Library of Congress Control Number: 2007908792

ISBN-10: 0-9801431-0-1
ISBN-13: 978-0-9801431-0-2

Table of Contents

Everything You Should and Need to Know
Definition ◆ Why Under diagnosed ◆ Scientific Diagnosis ◆
Psychosocial Impact ◆ Three Forms of Menopause ◆
Mood Swings ◆ Divorce During Menopause ◆ Case Studies ◆
Cardiovascular Health During Menopause ◆ Metabolic Concerns
During Menopause ◆ Osteoporosis and Osteopenia During
Menopause ◆ Pellet Hormone Delivery System ◆ SottoPelle Society
◆ Monitoring Hormone Therapy During Menopause ◆
Case Studies

Is There Really Such a Thing As Male Menopause?
Definition of Andropause ◆ Decrease in Androgens ◆ Symptoms
of Andropause ◆ When Does Andropause Occur? ◆ How Is
Andropause Diagnosed? ◆ Sex Binding Hormone Globulin ◆
Bioavailable Testosterone ◆ Low Testosterone Level ◆ Physical and
Intellectual Alterations During Andropause ◆ Hormonal
Replacement for Men ◆ Case Studies

Foreword

Symptomatic menopause, as anyone who has had the experience knows, is extremely unbearable in every aspect. Fortunately, there is finally relief for the healthy female with normal breasts.

Personally, I had all the symptoms: mental fog, hot flashes, inability to concentrate, insomnia, thinning hair, breast pain, dry skin and more. Pellet therapy has been thoroughly tested and has been available since 1939 in the United States. Over five years ago, I heard Dr. Gino Tutera explain the benefits of equivalent hormone replacement therapy and as both a physician and a patient, I decided to give it a try.

Pellet therapy is the only form of hormone replacement therapy that is biologically, physiologically, medically and pharmacologically sound. It is a form of hormone replacement therapy that best mimics your own natural hormone release from the ovaries. It is directly absorbed into the bloodstream; it is not altered by the liver as when you take pills—or unreliably absorbed through the skin, as with creams.

Four hours after my first pellet injection, the mental fog cleared. Thirty hours later, I had no more hot flashes; my energy returned; I could finally sleep through the night; and had enough energy left over to exercise and lose weight. I was NORMAL again!

I regained my life. Thanks to Dr. Tutera and this marvelous medical breakthrough, I feel like I'm thirty again—and I love it!—all thanks to pellet therapy.

As a breast surgeon, I both faithfully use and recommend pellet therapy to my patients who have normal, healthy breasts and are trying unsuccessfully to cope with those agonizing menopausal symptoms. It is truly the only natural therapy that makes good medical sense.

—Nedra J. Harrison, MD FACS
Breast Cancer Surgeon

Acknowledgements

To my loving wife Carolann, thank you so much for all your help and encouragement. Without your loving and gentle guidance, I would not be where I am. Without you this book would never have been completed. To my son Adam, thank you for your love and support. Thanks to my office staff for allowing me the time to work on this book! You are the best staff anyone could have! To Carol P., thanks for her support on the technical assistance! To John Robinson, NMD, my thanks for his contribution to the thyroid section of the book. Thanks to K Bell, whose poem, I hope, provides hope and insight for others!

And finally, my thanks to all the patients I have seen in the past, whose kind words stimulate me to continue doing what I do. Thank you for allowing me to enhance your lives!

Please enjoy this wonderful poem that I think says it better than I can.

I Got Those Hormone Blues

There I was popping those daily pills
When along came Dr. Tutera to save me from the aging & PMS ills

A "poke" every few months I get
And away go the headaches and the "gritch"

No night sweats, no sleepless nights
And oh baby, how I hold my loved one tight

The sex is GGGRRRRREEEAAATTTT
And so much more energy—never again late

But there is more to the story than meets the eye
With Dr. Tutera, less and less I cry

The pellets help keep me regulated day and night
Oh how they ease my mind, all right

No pill to pop, no cream to rub
Just a visit to Doc and I purr like a cub

So make that call today—without delay
Before you know it—you'll feel great like Kay.

Author: Kay "K" Bell

Introduction

All Things Possible

I doubt there is a man or woman among us who at one time or another hasn't asked themselves what they can do to look better, feel better, have more vitality, enjoy the same bounce they once did, and feel more in control of the symptoms associated with the aging process. Someone once said, "You can't control the wind, but you can control the sails." I do agree completely with this philosophy and it is for this reason I have written this book—I want to show you how you can manage the hormonal changes that will inevitably happen as we age, without compromising quality of life.

Can you remember what it felt like to be thirty? Your libido and sex drive were high. You didn't suffer from osteoporosis, heart disease or cancer. Why? Because your body chemistry was in balance and protected you.

As we age, we begin to lose the ability to produce those same levels of estrogen and testosterone. Optimum health is replaced with a host of age-related health problems. And we lose the vigor and energy for life we once had. And how many times have you heard the words, "you just have to accept it"?

The truth is nobody wants to become old or feel old. If you could change the way you age and just slow it down and keep feeling great—would you do it? Sure you would, especially if the method was medically safe, with rare side effects and successfully used by scores of others since the 1930s.

Don't be surprised if the pellet hormone delivery system helps you feel and look younger and you sense the return of emotional and physical well-being. Many years ago, women thought they had the remedy to maintain some youthful feeling while aging—the magic pill, as it was then known—synthetic hormone replacement therapy (HRT). It was touted as the wonder drug for women who had never had a hysterectomy who were approaching menopause or who were in menopause. Well, as we all know, that theory came to a screeching halt after the news in 2002 that the National Institutes of Health had halted the WHI trial because that combination drug, Prempro,[1] was found to be associated with a significant increase in the relative risk of breast cancer as well as significant increases in the relative risk of heart attack, stroke, and venous thrombosis. There is no question that this sudden occurrence caused women everywhere to be shattered, physicians were left floundering for an alternative and men were in disbelief over the trauma medicine had created for their wives. When the disheartening news was released in 2002, the OB/GYN world was thrown into a spiral that has yet to recover. Because the news blackened the use of all HRT therapy, most women are afraid to discuss the use of any hormonal therapy at all when in reality, there are options that are much safer than synthetic hormones and much easier to administer. Throughout my career as a practicing OB/GYN physician, I have focused more and more in the area of hormonal imbalance. And, I have been able to offer a safer option to women who are experiencing the discomforts of menopause, as well as men who are experiencing the discomforts of the male menopause, andropause.

Throughout my many years as a practicing OB/GYN physician, I have focused much of my practice on the treatment of hormonal imbalance and equivalent options. It is unfortunate that so few physicians in the United States are aware of the options that exist for the treatment of hormonal imbalance. Through this book I hope to improve awareness of these therapy options so that more physicians can offer this treatment and more patients will seek out physicians who understand the difference type of hormonal therapy that may be available to them.

Please enjoy reading this book as much as I enjoyed writing it. And, remember, you do have an option.

—Gino Tutera, MD

When hormone deficiency, caused by normal aging and menopause in women or andropause (male menopause) in men is diagnosed, an effective therapy is necessary if hormonal balance within the body is to be restored and relief from discomfort and symptoms is to be realized. Individualized hormone replacement therapy, through the use of the Pellet Hormone Delivery System (PHDS), is precise, personal, effective, consistent, reproducible, economical, reliable, and safe. Research shows that the uniqueness of this delivery system is an effective way to restore a balanced physiologic state. Studies have also repeatedly shown that using the Pellet Hormone Delivery System (PHDS) for hormone replacement outperforms all other equivalent methods of release.[2] Pills, creams, and patches do not deliver consistent levels of hormones to your system with the same confidence that the PHDS does.

Living with symptoms related to hormonal problems associated with aging, surgery, and related deficiencies is not the way to enjoy life and it doesn't have to be that way for anyone. For these reasons, I have written this book to help each of you gain a better understanding of what hormonal imbalance can do to you and to your quality of life. I hope to show you how you can bring your life back into balance through hormone therapy with the PHDS. You'll be able to eliminate the statement, "You'll just have to live with it" from the vocabulary of hormone replacement therapy so you can get on with your life the way you want it to be.

This book may also serve as an aid to physicians to help them to better understand their options for treating hormonal imbalance and encourage them to move beyond traditional, out-dated treatments for HRT. I will discuss PHDS in greater detail in later chapters within this book, provide case studies of some of my patients, and show that it is a well-researched therapy which has produced remarkable results for more than one thousand of my own patients over the last ten years and has been documented or researched in medical journals since 1938.[3] PHDS is currently used in England, Australia and other countries with great success, and has been thus used since 1939 in the United States.

In 2002, the National Institutes of Health halted the Prempro Women's Health Initiative (WHI) trial because the estrogen/progesterone combination was shown to be associated with a significant increase in the relative risk of breast cancer as well as a significant increase in the relative risk of heart attack, stroke, and venous thrombosis.[1] The stoppage of the study caused shock waves throughout our society because it demonstrated that oral conjugated estrogen, estrogen removed from horse urine, such as Premarin™, especially when coupled with synthetic progesterone (i.e., Premarin™, Provera™, Prempro™, Premphase™) caused a slight increase in the rate of breast cancer cases developing in the study group. Women who heard the news immediately called their physicians to ask what to do. In most cases, I believe the physicians asked them to stop taking the hormone replacement therapy until more understanding of the situation was realized.

The misinterpretation of the WHI study conclusion was the implication that ALL estrogen caused the same problems. *This is not the case at all.* Oral conjugated estrogen (Premarin™, etc.) is horse estrogen and is as different from human estrogen as night is to day. This would be comparable to saying that because one cosmetic company produces a bad mascara that all mascaras are bad for you.

As you read this book, you will see that the estrogen therapy discussed here is equivalent, which means it is exactly like that which the human body produces and will not cause any of the problems that horse estrogen or synthetic estrogen may cause. Pellet equivalent hormone therapy has shown positive research results since 1938 [3] and many papers providing these data have been published in respected international medical journals since that time. PHDS therapy was originally created specifically for women who had their ovaries removed. In fact, this form of therapy has been employed by different physicians in the Department of Endocrinology and Reproductive Endocrinology at the University of Georgia College of Medicine since 1939 and is still presently being utilized.[4,5]

Throughout my thirty plus years of practicing obstetrics and gynecology medicine, I have read, seen, and heard many opinions on hormonal therapy as a treatment for menopause, andropause (male menopause), and Post Menopausal Syndrome. While the topic of hormonal therapy continues to be confusing for the general public as well as the medical world, I believe I can help to eliminate most of the confusion and shed some light on a clearer path to maintaining hormonal balance and general well-being for women and men alike.

From the beginning of my medical career, I have maintained a keen interest in endocrinology, and, I continue to study within this therapeutic area today. While completing my residency in 1974, I initiated, wrote, and published a detailed research paper on the insulin levels in the amniotic fluid of diabetic pregnant women. During the course of this research, I became very interested in the human endocrine system, and I continue to follow current research and treatments in endocrinology today.

Don't let the words hormone replacement therapy scare you. This discussion is not about synthetic or horse hormones (pharmaceuticals), or even natural hormones (merely made from plants) that are not biologically equivalent. This discussion is about biologically equivalent hormones which are one hundred percent equivalent to those hormones created by the human body. Yes, they are made from botanicals, but, unlike the other natural hormones, they possess the equivalent biological structure and ensure exactly the same action as human hormones do.

For decades women and men have experienced the astounding benefits of biologically equivalent hormones for natural hormone replacement—that is, equivalent pellet therapy. In study after study, researchers have reported in highly respected medical journals how the use of equivalent estrogen and testosterone has positively impacted diseases such as osteoporosis, prostate cancer, and HIV.

With so much negative research surrounding pharmaceutical hormones, doesn't it make better sense to give your body what it recognizes and flourishes with? Of course it does. When research has proven that equivalent testosterone and estrogen pellets show no evidence of side effects, they are the obvious healthful choice.

Menopause and andropause do not have to mean the end of a happy, healthy, vivacious life. With the PHDS for equivalent hormones, you can achieve the balance of estrogen and testosterone your body needs to maintain optimum health. equivalent hormones replenish what is lost in the aging process, using the equivalent hormones your body used to create when you were healthy and in your prime—not synthetic pharmaceuticals.

Don't be surprised if your symptoms disappear—the fatigue goes away, along with those annoying hot flashes; your libido or sex drive improves; erectile dysfunction diminishes. You just have to believe how great you will feel using the PHDS for equivalent hormone therapy.

It is my intention, that after reading this book you will be better informed and able to ask more direct questions and seek more complete and satisfying answers from your physician. You will possess a deeper and clearer understanding of hormonal imbalance and what can be done to correct it. You will look into your crystal ball and see that your well-being is secure, your sex drive will be better, and many of those annoying side effects associated with menopause and andropause will be diminished.

Chapter 1

Understanding Menopause

"Education is the best provision for the journey to old age."
—Aristotle

When I ask patients to give me a definition of menopause, a variety of answers come back to me. The most common definition I hear is, "When you get hot flashes," followed by, "Not having a period for over a year." The fact is that most gynecologists and endocrinologists would agree that not having a period for a year is the definition of menopause. But in truth, menopause is often under diagnosed because of the failure of physicians to apply a scientific method for diagnosis. Scientifically, a diagnosis of the menopause needs to be stated quite simply: "A woman is in menopause when the level of follicle stimulating hormone (FSH), a pituitary hormone, reaches a level greater than twenty-three miu/ml, whether she is menstruating or not menstruating. In general, perimenopause or menopause transition begins when a woman is in her forties, with a mean age of forty-seven and a half years and an average duration of four to eight years. Menopause usually occurs at a mean age of fifty-one and two tenths years. Reproductive aging may occur as early as ten years prior to menopause and is evidenced by a rising follicle-stimulating hormone (FSH) level in the early follicular phase of the cycle and a decrease in inhibin B.[6] For several years, women in perimenopause may face marked biological variability, with subsequent endocrinologic and clinical changes. The mechanism by which neuroregulatory changes modulate the transition to menopause is still largely unknown. [6,7]

The interaction between these hormonal changes, the subsequent onset of menopause-related clinical symptoms, and the emergence of mood symptoms and cognitive deficits constitute a complex puzzle.[6] In the United States, more than one point three million women are expected to reach menopause every year. Dr. Claudio Soares described the relation between menopause and mood disturbance in a recent article[6] in this way: "During the menopausal transition, women may experience vasomotor symptoms and increased sexual dysfunction, as well as depressive symptoms, leading to a significant psychosocial impairment." There are many women suffering the ravages of menopause, and many continue to go untreated. You might find it surprising to know that the number of women who are still menstruating and in menopause is not an insignificant one. Although many women may be asymptomatic, estrogen deficiency is associated with hot flashes, severe sweating, insomnia, and vaginal dryness and discomfort in up to eighty-five percent of menopausal women. Hormone therapy (HT) is the most effective intervention for management of these quality-of-life symptoms.[8]

If you are going through menopause or perimenopause, you may still be worried about what your life is going to look like after it's all over. You are probably a little scared about how your body will feel, how your mood will be, and whether or not you will be able to enjoy life in the same way. Well, put your fears to rest, because life after menopause can be quite enjoyable.

While we all refer to this change of life in one lump term as menopause, there are actually several different forms of menopause: premature ovary failure

(POF), surgical menopause, and natural menopause. All three impose risks of earlier development of heart disease, bone loss, brain dysfunction (dementia), musculoskeletal dysfunction, and loss of sexual desire and function.[8]

> *"Put your fears away, life after menopause can be quite enjoyable."*

Premature Ovarian Failure (POF) is actually the onset of menopause before age forty, diagnosed in women when ovarian function stops. There are serious consequences to POF other than infertility, and sadly many physicians are not fully aware of this fact. With POF, up to fifty percent of patients may ovulate once in any given year and five percent to ten percent of patients may become pregnant, leading to a theory that there is a follicular dysfunction rather than complete ovarian failure. Women with POF go through the same loss of estrogen as menopausal women in their fifties, but usually faster or suddenly, as do women who have surgery to remove their ovaries. In many cases, the estrogen loss in POF is even before these women have had the full benefits of estrogen in their lives, such as building maximal bone mass.

The loss of estrogen puts women at increased risk for this dysfunction, osteoporosis, heart disease, colon cancer, Alzheimer's disease, tooth loss, impaired vision, Parkinson's disease and diabetes. The longer women are without the protection of their own estrogen, the greater their risk for serious health consequences of these conditions.[9]

Unfortunately, the diagnosis of POF is often delayed because many physicians do not always consider this to be a working differential diagnosis. It may take visits to several physicians, over a long period of time, before the diagnosis is recognized. In actuality, a simple blood test of hormonal therapy measuring the Follicle Stimulating Hormone (FSH) level will confirm the diagnosis when the FSH level is over twenty-five miu/ml, not just over forty miu/ml on two occasions over a four week period.[9] Because POF is most often not scientifically diagnosed, women suffering from this are left to go untreated. In actual practice, if physicians were to adhere to the clear definition of menopause: hot flashes, irritability, etc., and an elevation of the FSH level, the women suffering premature menopause would not be ignored or incorrectly treated. Premature menopause can occur at any age and is more common than one might think. It is not usually suspected because the average age for menopause to begin is fifty-one. Perhaps, the definition of premature menopause should be stated to be the development of menopausal symptoms, the loss of normal estrogen levels, the elevation of the hormone of FSH above 25—and not the complete loss of menstrual periods for twelve months.

Premature menopause may result from a variety of causes. Certain gynecological and obstetrical conditions can result in premature menopause such as Sheehan's syndrome, endometriosis, or sudden failure of the ovaries, termed premature ovarian failure (POF). There are chromosomal and genetic causes such as Turner's syndrome. Medical conditions that can lead to premature menopause are systemic lupus, insulin dependant diabetes, kidney disease and failure, and certain liver diseases. Radiation of the abdomen and pelvis to treat malignant disease can also cause premature menopause, as can the chemotherapy regimens for the treatment of cancer.

CASE STUDY

Cheryl, a thirty-nine-year-old female, presented to me with complaints of inability to sleep, increased anxiety, hot flashes, and cold sweats occurring at night for over twelve months, as well as a complaint of having no sex drive for the past two years. Her period was still occurring every six to eight weeks. Her gynecologist at the time felt that she was suffering from anxiety and depression and prescribed Zoloft for these symptoms. Her symptoms did improve, but she knew she wasn't depressed. She had a great marriage and family and had no real problems at home. Her hot flashes and anxiety, although better, continued as did her low sex drive and low energy level.

When I first saw Cheryl in my clinic, I immediately obtained a basic hormone profile blood test including a measure of the pituitary hormone FSH. Her test results showed that she had an elevated FSH to over forty, which is diagnostic of menopause, as well as a low estrogen and testos-

terone levels near zero. Based on these test results, I instituted estrogen and testosterone HRT via PHDS. Six weeks after the introduction of this therapy, Cheryl's FSH was down to eighteen and her hormone levels of estrogen and testosterone were completely normal. Her words to me were, **"I'm my old self again, thank you for giving me back my life. I'm no longer taking any antidepressant medication and once again I feel like a normal woman. P.S., my husband really thanks you."**

Surgical menopause is more easily defined than POF; however, it is just as severe. Surgical menopause begins when both ovaries are removed and estrogen and testosterone productions are completely eliminated except for a tiny amount of each that comes from the adrenal glands. A woman who has had her uterus removed or the uterus and one ovary removed and then develops menopausal symptoms and changes in her estrogen and FSH levels should also be included in this category because the effects are identical. The changes that surgery can impose on any residual ovarian tissue can cause it to fail and place the patient immediately in menopause, regardless of her chronological age.

While premature menopause or POF is the gradual development of menopausal symptoms at an early age, post menopausal ovaries can still produce testosterone and the menopausal symptoms may develop in a much more gradual manner. In surgical menopause there are substantial and immediate drops in estrogen and testosterone production within forty-eight hours of ovarian removal. Any hormones produced by the ovaries at the time of removal may persist for a short period of time, but usually are gone within that two-day period.

The recognition of the differences between premature menopause and surgical menopause by physicians is essential because the effects on brain, muscle, bone, heart, and metabolism for women can be substantial and dangerous. The denial of estrogen and testosterone to the brain will most definitely result in very labile emotions since the loss of hormones causes decreased serotonin production. Labile emotions result in more anxiety, irritability, sleep disturbances, anger, sadness, and depression. Low estrogen levels affect mood.

As noted author and lecturer, Colette Dowling, M.S.W. related,[46] **"From early fetal life, hormone receptors are present in the hypothalamus of the brain. It is here that they begin organizing brain circuitry, setting the stage for puberty, regulating subsequent adult sexual behavior, and controlling the frequency and intensity of emotional disorders. Research in neuroendocrinology has much to tell us about the pre-menopausal malaise that used to be thought the result of women's sadness over the loss of reproductive function. Now it's known that the mood and cognitive changes some women experience during perimenopause are physical in origin." Low estrogen affects mood. In order to produce serotonin the brain needs estrogen. There are estrogen receptors in various organs throughout the body, the brain included. That's why estrogen loss produces so many different bodily symptoms—loss of skin elasticity, bone shrinkage, mood and cognitive decline.**

When estrogen levels rise, on the other hand, as they do in the first week of menses, their overall effect is to increase the amount of serotonin available in the spaces between the brain's nerve cells. That improves mood. Within the brain, estrogen may in fact act as a natural antidepressant and mood stabilizer. Therefore, it is essential that a woman suffering from POF or surgical menopause be treated by a physician with whom she can develop a trusting relationship who can understand all of the ramifications of the disease and be willing and able to meet her endocrine and emotional needs.

The musculoskeletal system is also adversely affected by the loss of estrogen and testosterone which can lead to the early development of muscle atrophy, osteopenia, osteoporosis, and pain in the muscles and joints. We do expect these difficulties as we age, but we do not expect them to happen during our thirties and forties as will commonly happen with premature menopause and surgical menopause.

The emergence of data supporting the theory that fluctuations in estrogen levels may profoundly influence mood supports the existence of such a climacteric syndrome before the final cessation of periods. Changes in the pattern of ovarian hormone secretion are often associated with the development of depression.[10] How many marriages and relationships have suffered or failed because of these changes? In fact, according to AARP statistics, more than fifty percent of divorces initiated by women occur after the age of fifty. The other half are usually initiated by men who can no longer tolerate the behaviors that hormonal losses induce in the woman they love. Depression and mood swings create an unpleasant environment in the home and if they are not managed, can cause a split in a marriage or relationship.

Women who lose their ability to produce serotonin, a neurotransmitter derived from tryptophan that is involved in sleep, depression, memory, and other neurological processes, are less likely to cope with stress rationally and more than likely will become volatile, explosive, and irrational. This most certainly can have serious adverse impact on personal and business relationships. I have numerous patients who have lost their marriages, jobs, and relationships with friends and family because of their hormonal changes. The loss of both ovarian hormones, estrogen and testosterone, also causes a decrease in a transmitter substance in the brain called acetylcholine, which allows rapid transmission of impulses from one nerve cell to another. If hormones are absent, less acetylcholine is produced and the brain no longer can function as it once did. One of the many important focuses of testosterone is to help the brain to stay focused and promote the retention of the ability to concentrate and maintain a normal attention span. Primary complaints I often hear are, "I can't think clearly," and "I wonder if I have Attention Deficit Disorder (ADD)," or "I wonder if I have early Alzheimer's disease." Short-term memory is also adversely affected by loss of ovarian hormones. This places an underlying fear in patients that something ominous such as Alzheimer's or dementia is beginning. When a patient in her thirties experiences these effects, she is terrified.

CASE STUDY

Dana, a thirty-five-year-old woman real estate agent, presented to me because her physician told her the "fuzzy thinking and poor memory" were all related to stress and that she should try to work through her problems with exercise and stress reduction. The problem was she was always so tired that she was unable to exercise. She had asked her previous physician to run a hormone panel blood test to see if her hormones were low, and he refused by telling her she was "young and healthy, and the tests were unreliable anyway."

When Dana came to my clinic, I ordered a hormone panel blood test for her and the results showed that her testosterone level was zero. I immediately began Dana on testosterone therapy via the PHDS. Four weeks after the testosterone therapy began, Dana told me, "I can think again and my energy level is so good. I can exercise without feeling completely exhausted."

According to the American Association of Clinical Endocrinologists Medical Guidelines for Clinical Practice for the Diagnosis and Treatment of Menopause, coronary artery disease (CAD) is the leading cause of death in postmenopausal women. Scientific studies have demonstrated that "estrogen has direct antiatherogenic effects in the coronary arteries at a molecular level and prevents the formation of atheromatous fat plaques in the oophorectomized model in humans."[11] A woman's cardiovascular health is dependant on the presence of estrogen. When she is deprived of estrogen, her risk of coronary heart disease (CHD) or stroke increases at a much younger age. This risk of CHD is extremely dangerous in women who have a family history of heart disease or have diabetes. Lack of awareness about the significant effects on the cardiovascular system of women who are afflicted with premature or surgical menopause is in effect shortening their life span. Premature menopause or surgical menopause can also cause adverse effects on serum cholesterol, and triglycerides and further promote the acceleration of plaque formation in the arteries and premature aging of the cardiovascular system.

The metabolic effects of testosterone on the muscle help to induce a stabilization of blood sugar (glucose) and its rapid utilization by the muscle. Testosterone allows the body to use glucose more effectively, thereby allowing the body to sustain normal insulin levels. If on the other hand, the muscle takes up the glucose too slowly, blood sugar will rise and cause increased fat deposition. This leads to a condition termed insulin resistance, which can lead to high blood pressure, obesity, and the condition called "metabolic syndrome", or Type II diabetes. Metabolic Syndrome (MS) was once called Syndrome X, but now has been shown to be a primary cause of menopausal middle (fat deposited around the waist and hips) in women and "beer gut "in men. MS can lead to high cholesterol, obesity, and high blood pressure. Is it any wonder then that so many women gain fifteen to twenty-five pounds after premature menopause or especially, surgical menopause? Typically, a healthcare provider will tell a woman, "You are just eating too much and not exercising enough." In fact, women who undergo surgical menopause or develop premature menopause will usually gain weight— which is nearly impossible to lose without the institution of appropriate hormone therapy. The proper therapy really must be the recreation of the normal physiologic levels of estrogen and testosterone, which can only be done through the use of biologically equivalent hormones delivered by the Pellet Hormone Delivery System.

Osteopenia and osteoporosis are significantly increased in women suffering from premature menopause and surgical menopause, because these women are not monitored or diagnosed properly. The women who suffer through these types of menopause are usually initially given hormones with no monitoring of blood levels of hormones or bone break-down factors. Traditionally, bone density studies are not done at an early age to check for the development of osteopenia or osteoporosis. The number of women that I see with problems such as these who have premature menopause or surgical menopause has increased quite dramatically over the ones who have had bone density studies where diagnosis is made and treatment is begun. The effect on improving bone density with the use of hormonal pellets is substantial. Studies have show that the use of equivalent hormone pellets increases the bone density by eight point three per cent.[12] This percentage may be better than what is seen with the oral non hormonal osteoporosis medications.

CASE STUDIES

CarolAnn, my wife, was diagnosed with osteoporosis at forty-three years of age. Her hormone profile demonstrated she was in menopause and possessed low estrogen and testosterone levels, even though she was still menstruating regularly. She had occasional "warm feelings" and difficulty sleeping, but since she was only forty-three, she was told by her physician at the time it was due to her heavy work load—taking care of her family and managing her business. Her Dexa Scan II report, an instrument used to diagnose osteoporosis, revealed osteoporosis of the spine. She was placed on therapy of estradiol and testosterone pellets. Within six months from the start of therapy, her bone density was normal for a woman her age.

Robert, a seventy-three-year-old male, was being treated for osteoporosis with a weekly medication that he had been on for the past three years, during which time his osteoporosis never improved. His T. Value, an estimation of bone density, was minus three point seven (any value higher than minus two point five indicates osteoporosis). His value indicated bones as strong as soda crackers and high fracture risk. He wasn't improving because his testosterone was so low. After receiving testosterone pellets, his testosterone was raised to the level of a thirty-year-old man. He stopped his weekly osteoporosis medicine after six months, and after fourteen months his T. Value had decreased to minus one point one which is above normal for anyone of seventy-three years. It is now three years after starting his therapy on testosterone pellets, and his bone density remains normal. He has much greater muscle mass which has helped to improve his mobility and as a result, has improved his quality of life. His prostate is smaller and his PSA (prostate cancer test) remains excellent.

The lack of awareness within the medical community of the fact that there are three types of menopause, or the ability to recognize a differential diagnosis for each of the different types of menopause places a significant risk on those younger women suffering with premature menopause or surgical menopause. As previously discussed, these women are very often ignored or inappropriately treated. Their cardiovascular health, cerebral health, metabolic balance, and skeletal health are usually taken for granted because of their youth. There is no excuse today for a young woman in her thirties or forties to have the physiologic age of a fifty- to seventy-year-old person, and it certainly is time that healthcare providers recognized this fact. Other healthcare providers are frequently astonished when they are shown the lab work completed in our clinics that reveals the level of deficiency of hormones in these women. All healthcare professionals must become aware of the significant barriers to good health and well-being faced by these women and attempt to provide the necessary care and guidance.

The treatment of premature menopausal and/or surgical menopausal women appears to remain in the dark ages. Physicians fail to realize the absolute need to return these women to a "normal" physiologic state, not just get rid of their "hot flashes" and "dry vaginas," but to achieve hormonal balance and total well-being. The traditional oral, patch, or cream hormone can take care of some of these complaints, but women who have suffered premature menopause and surgical menopause require a much different therapy. They require higher levels of hormones delivered in a continuous manner. High amounts of oral, patch, and cream hormones may cause the development of abnormal clotting factors, high bad cholesterol, and breast disease.

Women who have developed premature menopause and/or surgical menopause need to have these hormones delivered in a manner that recreates the continuous flow of hormones that the ovaries previously produced within their bodies. The only form of hormone delivery that comes close is the PHDS, the only therapy of its type that can establish a normal physiologic dose of estrogen and testosterone that recreates a true ovarian environment.

SottoPelle® Therapy Society physicians are trained in the use of PHDS in the treatment of these specific groups of patients as well as natural menopause patients. The method of delivery of the equivalent hormone is more important than the type of hormone, because if the hormone is not constantly present the patient cannot have the normal physiologic state she once had. PHDS is the only system today that allows the body to control the release of the hormones over time. Premature menopause and surgical menopause cannot be corrected unless the body is returned to a normal physiologic state, and nothing in an oral, patch, or cream form can reproduce that. Unfortunately, physicians and healthcare providers do not follow blood hormone levels on patients who are receiving therapy because it is generally, if not universally, felt that hormone levels fluctuate too much to provide for an accurate estimation of adequate therapy, and only symptoms relief should be utilized.

Actually if the FSH is utilized to judge adequacy of estrogen levels in the body and not just the estrogen level itself, accurate monitoring of patients can be accomplished. The FSH is as effective in diagnosing the adequacy of estrogen therapy as a TSH is in diagnosing thyroid hormone excess or deficiency. They both will diagnose a normal or abnormal state of their respective hormones. The FSH and TSH are only easily and accurately measured by using blood. In fact, the recent use of saliva testing is useless since it cannot detect these hormones.

The complete and proper treatments for premature menopause and surgical menopause are so important in restoring a normal healthy physiologic state that saliva testing, being done today, needs to be abandoned and appropriate blood studies completed and properly interpreted. The interpretation of these studies is further discussed within later chapters of this book.

Chapter 2

Andropause— the Decline of Testosterone

"The trick is growing up without growing old."
—Casey Stengel

By now, you must be pretty well versed on menopause and all of the attending miseries that can go with it—both big and small. But what do you know about male andropause? If you're like most people, probably very little. Or maybe you don't know anything about it at all. Let's begin by answering a few basic questions.

What is Andropause?
In a word, *andropause* is the male version of *menopause*. It is caused by the same thing a woman experiences—a decline in hormone production. For a man this means that over time his body will manufacture less and less testosterone. Surprisingly, the decline begins at around the age of thirty. Beyond that age, male hormone levels drop by approximately ten percent every decade. By the time a man is between forty and fifty-five

13

years of age, his testosterone levels will drop appreciably and signal the onset of andropause. Since testosterone is central to a man's well-being, he will often experience a variety of disturbing physical and emotional changes. These might include things like chronic fatigue, loss of energy, low sex drive, diminished physical agility and increased belly fat.

Why Haven't We Heard More About Andropause?

A big reason andropause has not made the front page headlines is the social stigma attached to issues of masculinity. (The same is also true of femininity.) And no man wants to hear that what makes him a man—i.e., his testosterone—is not up to snuff. In years past when men experienced a physical decline or emotional changes, they assumed that it was some kind of mid-life crisis thing. And their doctors most often encouraged them to accept their plight because they weren't 'spring chickens' anymore. So, things like hair loss, paunchiness, or erectile dysfunction were either not talked about or dismissed as something you couldn't do anything about. You just had to live with it.

Since the 1940s, however, there has been far more research on the human body and the importance of hormones in overall health. Today we know that testosterone deficiency can be linked to osteoporosis, heart disease, moodiness, depression, low energy levels, sexual dysfunction, and other problems that crop up in later life.

When Does Andropause Occur?

Most men will experience andropause between the ages of forty and fifty-five, at which time they can be said to be testosterone deficient. Unlike a woman, a man doesn't have a clear-cut indication like the cessation of menstruation to mark the arrival of andropause. Although a decline in testosterone levels will occur in virtually all men as they age, there is no way to predict who will experience andropausal symptoms severe enough to seek medical help. Each man's symptoms vary as does the age at which those symptoms occur. Jed Diamond, author of the book *Male Menopause*, reports that as many as twenty-five million males between ages forty and fifty-five are experiencing some degree of male menopause today. As shocking as these figures may seem to us, physicians are becoming more and more aware of andropause and beginning to scientifically diagnose it instead of simply offering a prescription for an undiagnosed disease that doesn't address the basic problem.

Although the first study on male andropause was published in the *Journal of the American Medical Association* in the mid-1940s, it's only recently that the United States medical community noticed this condition, stated Dr. Adrian Dobs, an endocrinologist and associate professor of medicine at the Johns Hopkins School of Medicine.

How Is Andropause Diagnosed?

In the past, a man suffering from symptoms of andropause was treated for a specific medical condition, such as depression. He was prescribed an antidepressant and left his doctor's office thinking his conditions was properly treated. We know that by treating andropause this way, the other symptoms such as loss of libido were not treated by the antidepressant and in fact were probably exaggerated.

When you go to your doctor for an annual exam, it's a good time to discuss any symptoms you may be having and request blood tests to measure your hormone levels. It is important that both free testosterone and total testosterone are tested, along with other hormones and indicators of your overall state of health. The results of those tests may suggest that your body is not producing adequate levels of hormone for optimum health and you have entered andropause. Today we know that just because we aren't "spring chickens" doesn't mean that we have to accept the aging-related decline in health that our fathers and grandfathers once did. Medical science has changed everything.

The truth is you do _not_ have to live with it! There is strong evidence that testosterone is very important to maintaining optimum health in both men and women. Studies suggest that testosterone directly affects muscle development, fat levels, bone mass, many different parts of the brain, moods, depression, energy levels, ability to have orgasms, heart health and ability to sleep. Testosterone replacement therapy continues to receive a great deal of medical support and the benefits are well documented in a multitude of clinical trials, dating back as far as the 1940s.

The negative press you've seen on testosterone is based solely on studies performed using *pharmaceutical testosterone* and *anabolic steroids*. Biologically equivalent testosterone pellets are free of the serious side effects associated with those synthetics. Research continues to support the use of all-natural, *biologically equivalent testosterone* in healthful doses, especially when pellet therapy is used. Remember, pellet therapy is the only delivery system capable of delivering those healthful doses twenty-four/seven, directly into the bloodstream, bypassing the liver. It has time and again demonstrated the ability to support good health, slow the aging process and readily alleviate andropause-related symptoms. Who do you think about first when you hear the word hormone? For most of us, it is a woman—more specifically, a woman and menopause. Age-related hormonal decline has been mainly in women, but we are beginning to see more and more scientific investigation into hormonal changes in the aging male. Current medical research now defines a male equivalent to menopause as andropause.

Aging is accompanied by gradual but progressive reductions in the secretion of testosterone and growth hormone in men.[13] Men lose approximately one percent of their testosterone and two point five percent of their DHEA per year beginning at age thirty. The impact of decreasing androgens is known as andropause, also called "male menopause" or ADAM—Androgen Decline in the Aging Male. It is a normal part of aging, although for some men it is accompanied by a gradual and undesired decline in their sexuality, mood and overall energy. Sometimes it can even expose men to more serious health risks.

On or about age thirty, testosterone levels in men drop by about ten percent every decade. At the same time, another factor in the body called Sex Binding Hormone Globulin, or SHBG, is increasing. SHBG traps much of the testosterone that is still circulating and makes it unavailable to exert its effects in the body's tissues. What's left does the beneficial work and is known as "bioavailable" testosterone.

"Andropause is associated with low (bioavailable) testosterone levels, which every man experiences, but some men's levels dip lower than others. And when this happens, this group of men can experience andropausal symptoms that can impact their quality of life and may expose them to other, longer-term risks of low-testosterone. It is estimated that thirty percent of men in their fifties will have testosterone levels low enough to be causing symptoms. Andropause is often characterized by a variety of physical and intellectual alterations that include:"[14]

- Decreased sexual desire and increased erectile dysfunction
- Changes in mood associated with fatigue, depression and anger with concomitant decreases in intellectual activity and spatial orientation ability
- Decreased lean body mass with associated diminution in muscle volume and strength accompanied by increases in visceral fat
- Decreased body hair and skin alterations such as increases in facial wrinkling
- Decreased bone mineral density resulting in osteoporosis

Dr. Robert Tan, an internationally recognized Geriatrician who specializes in aging andrology, describes andropause in this way: "Between the ages of fifty to seventy years, some men report symptoms such as erectile dysfunction (failure to achieve an erection), general tiredness, mood changes, night sweats and sometimes palpitations. Night sweats and palpitations occur because of an overactive autonomic system in response to falling testosterone levels." Dr. Tan further states, "I believe men want to be on hormonal replacement, and they need to hear from their doctors that it is safe and effective. Doctors have a responsibility to their patients as their practice is rooted on "evidence-based medicine." At this point, hormonal replacement for men should be considered on a case-by-case basis, depending on symptoms. Over the next decade or two, as more information is available, I do foresee that hormonal replacement will be more routine and perhaps replace some of the self-help regimens that men are experimenting with now."[27, 28]

Although andropause was first observed in the 1940s, our ability to diagnose it properly is still very poor. Sensitive tests for bioavailable testosterone weren't available until recently, so andropause has gone through a long period where it was underdiagnosed and undertreated. Now that men are living longer there is heightened interest in andropause, and this will help to advance medicine's approach to this important life stage.

The potential benefits of equivalent hormonal replacement therapy in aging men may include an increase in bone mineral density and reduction in fractures—a similar response to what is seen in postmenopausal women receiving estrogen replacement. Hormonal therapy delivered through the PHDS may also result in increases in lean body mass and possibly strength and a decrease in fat mass and potentially improves metabolic sensitivity. After hormonal treatment, men may also see an enhancement of libido and/or increased sexual drive and a reduction in fatigue with an increase in energy levels. The benefit to PHDS therapy for men as with women is the pellets deliver a continuous delivery of hormones based on the body's needs.

"In essence, hormonal replacement therapy for men reestablishes the sense of overall well-being, restores muscle mass and strength, increases energy, improves libido and erectile quality and promotes better mental clarity."

It bypasses the liver and thus avoids any additional complications. In essence, hormonal replacement therapy for men reestablishes the sense of overall well-being, restores muscle mass and strength, increases energy, improves libido and erectile quality and promotes mental clarity.

Studies suggest that testosterone directly impacts muscle development, fat levels, bone mass, many different parts of the brain, moods, depression, energy levels, ability to have orgasms, and ability to sleep. Anxiety and irritability are increased in both men and women who suffer from testosterone deficiency.

Steroids Are Not the Real Deal

Testosterone contains two parts: an anabolic part (for building muscle), and an androgenic part (for developing masculine traits and libido). Anabolic steroids are prescription drugs that mimic testosterone's muscle-building properties. Unfortunately, you've heard plenty about anabolic use in the sports world. Most physicians distrust these synthetics and the federal government regulates them, thanks to some unforgettably embarrassing Olympic moments.

Receiving equivalent testosterone is not the same as taking an anabolic. There are many positive studies that have been reported on equivalent testosterone replacement therapy for both men and women—especially in the pellet form that is used in PHDS Therapy.

The Testosterone Myths

It is true that excess testosterone can cause a variety of side effects. Too much is too much, and the body responds accordingly. This takes us back to what we have been saying about balance. It is a delicate act. If you take too much or use synthetic and chemically treated testosterone you can expect serious consequences—like hair loss, facial hair (in women), water retention, irritability, acne, headaches, joint stiffness, prostate problems and increased liver enzymes.

But don't let anyone talk you out of replacing what your body needs. You won't grow a mustache or go bald if you restore your testosterone to its formerly healthy levels. The endocrine system is a fantastic balanced system with exquisite feedback controls. When utilizing equivalent hormone in PHDS therapy, the body responds like it's business as usual. It merely replaces the normal amounts that it is used to   simple as that.

How Do You Know If You Are Experiencing Andropause?

The ADAM test (Androgen Deficiency in Aging Men) is a tool used to screen for symptoms of low testosterone in men over forty years of age. This is just a first step in assessing an unequivocal diagnosis of andropause. The questions below are just a few that might address some of the symptoms of andropause. There are many others that you may want to add to this list. Answer as many as you can and then discuss them with your physician.

- Are you experiencing a decreased sex drive?
  If yes, for how long?
- Are your erections as strong as they should be?
- How is your energy level lately? If you feel like you are lacking the energy you normally have, please describe.
- Has your height changed?
- How is your endurance during physical activities?
- Have you lost the athletic ability you have always had?
- Do you feel as though you have the same strength as you normally do?
- Have you lost the feeling of enjoying life?
- Do you feel sad or irritable more often than usual?
- Are you falling asleep earlier and earlier every night?
- How is your work performance? Is it deteriorating?

CASE STUDIES

Art, a sixty-five-year-old retired dentist, came to see me because he was feeling tired a good deal of the time, was not able to exercise regularly, had lost his sex drive, was experiencing erectile dysfunction and was noticing short term memory problems. His wife, who was also my patient, had previously experienced success with PHDS therapy and brought her husband to me for evaluation. His blood workup revealed a testosterone level of two hundred and a low level of free testosterone. He stated that his family doctor had looked at a copy of our lab work and told him that two hundred was normal for his age. He actually was below the normal range (two hundred fifty to one thousand), but his doctor's statement revealed a similar prejudice to one we often see in our office — the older the man is, the lower the testosterone he should have. In fact, I feel that men can become normal if they have testosterone levels between seven hundred and eleven hundred as they did in their thirties. He received testosterone by way of the PHDS, which brought his testosterone level up to nine hundred. His physician felt this was too high, but as Art stated, "I feel so young, I don't care what you say—this feels right for me." He's now been on this therapy for three years and hasn't had any problems. He has also changed his family physician.

John, a fifty-year-old gentleman, presented to me because he was feeling extreme fatigue, noticing loss of memory, poor muscle tone, and was experiencing poor recovery after regular exercise (from the past years). He also had a diminished sex drive. His laboratory blood test values indicated a low normal testosterone of three hundred twenty (two hundred fifty to eleven hundred is the range) and a low free testosterone level.

John received testosterone pellets by way of the PHDS and eight weeks later when we checked his testosterone level, it had risen to one thousand. He stated, "I feel so much better. My exercise is showing results and my energy is never better. My brain is working again and sex drive is as good as it was five years ago."

Note: John's case study is an example of how a man can have low normal levels of hormones and still be hormone deficient. His body, when at its best, was producing higher levels of testosterone and functioned better at higher testosterone levels. It is common practice for physicians to look at laboratory blood test values, and if they are in the range of normal, to believe that there is no indication for any therapy. Physicians must become more aware of the fact that men need to maintain the same levels of testosterone that they had when they were in their twenties and thirties if they are to feel vital, healthy, and maintain a normal quality of life. Low normal testosterone levels just won't do it!

If you are experiencing any of the symptoms described in this chapter and you want to regain your vitality and sense of well-being, speak with your physician about andropause and possible treatment with testosterone

PHDS therapy. Don't accept andropause; there are options for treatment.

Words to live by when it comes to andropause:
"Growing old is no more than a bad habit which a busy person has no time to form."
—Andre Maurois

Chapter 3

Hormone Imbalance— Identifying the Symptoms

"Living well is the best revenge."
—Anonymous

When your hormones are in balance, you know it. You look great, you feel terrific, you have plenty of energy and you sleep like a baby. Your immune system and your digestive system are in tiptop shape. This is your body's way of saying, "Hey, go ahead, relax and enjoy life—I'm feeling great."

It's only when you begin to age and your hormone levels take a dive that your world begins to feel less than friendly. You gain weight, you lose interest in sex, you aren't sleeping as well as you once did, you can't seem to think straight—the list goes on and on. You soon discover that getting older is not about getting better; it's about getting harder to stay better. Not only do you feel a lot less perky, more sluggish, and have less endurance, but you now have health issues to deal with. Pretty soon things like cardiovascular disease, high blood pressure, diabetes and osteoporosis show up and you have to stop your life to deal with them.

Didn't someone say these are the golden years? What is it about hormonal balance that can make such a "night and day" difference in our lives?

Hormonal Balance = Health

Hormones are your body's chemical messengers. They travel in your bloodstream to tissues or organs throughout the body. They work slowly, over time, and affect many different processes, including:

- Growth and development
- Metabolism—how your body gets energy from the foods you eat
- Sexual function
- Reproduction
- Mood

Hormones rejuvenate, regenerate, and restore. They may seem small, but they are very powerful. It takes only a small amount of a hormone to cause big changes in cells or even disturb the balance within your whole body. Too much or too little of a certain hormone can be very serious.

Ask any endocrinologist and he or she will tell you that hormonal balance equates to health. Our hormones give us life, intelligence, mood, drive, sexuality, physical and mental energy, and the desire to grow, learn and achieve. They are not in our body by mistake. They are there to allow us to function well and enjoy the world we live in.

Since our hormone-producing glands control our basic body functions such as metabolism, growth and sexual development, it is critical that the amount of hormone manufactured by each gland is carefully balanced. Too much or too little can have effects throughout the body and cause a variety of disorders.

Let's review some of the important hormones and look at how they work as a catalyst for specific functions within the body.

Estrogen

During a woman's childbearing years, which are generally her most healthful, her ovaries produce a balance of three important estrogens: estradiol, estriol and estrone. Estradiol is the predominant estrogen, produced in twice the amount of the other estrogens in the blood. To function at its best, a woman's body must maintain this ratio of two to one. If the ratio is altered, too much estrone is created. Estrone is a very strong breast stimulator. One reason women complain of breast tenderness with on oral estrogen is because the ratio is disturbed, resulting in excess estrone. With conjugated or synthetic estrogens, the ratio is actually reversed to an unhealthy one to two.

Estrogen is a powerful hormone that is found everywhere—in both men and women, in plants producing compounds with estrogen-like qualities (phytoestrogens), in environmental compounds (xenoestrogens) found in pesticides, meats or plastics, and in chemical estrogens made by pharmaceutical companies.

Strong evidence suggests that declining estrogen levels within a woman's body appear to be associated with reduction of muscle mass, increase in fat mass and a gradual weight increase.

Not All Estrogens Are Created Equal

Since 1930 over one hundred synthetic estrogens have been developed. Many are more potent than the natural estrogens. The cancer-producing and heart disease-promoting effects of these new compounds are only beginning to be recognized in humans. Thank goodness the number of doctors in favor of using biologically equivalent estrogen, which matches the body's own chemistry, is growing. Remember—what the media and even studies often refer to as 'estrogen' is not actually true estrogen. Synthetic compounds are not equivalent to what the body produces. So, when women hear that estrogen is bad for them, they don't realize they are hearing about the negative studies surrounding pharmaceuticals. And further, when women are made to fear their own estrogen, there is something terribly amiss in the land.

It is very troublesome to me that even in today's enlightened field of medicine, the medical schools do not place sufficient emphasis on how to properly diagnose and formulate a therapy program for the hormonal problems associated with menopause and andropause. Virtually no current physician-teaching programs that I know of make any mention of equivalent hormone therapy.

Too often I have heard both my male and female patients say, "I wish this would just go away." It is an amazing fact that men and women who suffer from hormonal difficulties have the same symptoms and complaints. These symptoms are due to estrogen and testosterone deficiencies for both sexes.

Please review the following lists and you may be surprised to see that many of the same symptoms describe both men and women.

Symptom	Women	Men
Anxiety	Yes	Yes
Irritability	Yes	Yes
Fatigue	Yes	Yes
Loss of Energy	Yes	Yes
Poor Mental Focus	Yes	Yes
Poor Concentration	Yes	Yes
Depression	Yes	Yes
Loss of Muscle Tone	Yes	Yes
Decreased Ability to Exercise	Yes	Yes
Prolonged Recovery After Exercise	Yes	Yes
No Physical Improvement With Exercise	Yes	Yes
Weight Gain in Spite of Exercise	Yes	Yes
Loss of Memory	Yes	Yes
Osteoporosis	Yes	Yes
Decreased Sexual Desire	Yes	Yes
Loss of Cardiac Protection	Yes	Yes
Higher Bad Cholesterol	Yes	Yes
Hot Flashes	Yes	No
Decreased Erectile Function	No	Yes
Night Sweats	Yes	No
Prostate Enlargement	No	Yes

With all the negative effects caused by estrogen and testosterone deficiency, wouldn't you want to find a way to make these symptoms go away? Unfortunately, these problems don't take care of themselves. Unless you take action and seek help, your overall well-being will continue to worsen. Hormonal balance cannot be achieved by guess work or with insufficient information.

You have probably come across people who say they don't have any of these problems, or that their problems "went away" by themselves. Yes, they may have had a decrease in the frequency and severity of their symptoms, but the more serious problems of heart attack, stroke, osteoporosis, depression, and loss of mental acuity all continue to worsen. Denial is a handy method we use all too often. We want to fix our problems ourselves, but there are issues that can be treated safely only through the use of hormonal treatment to restore balance, and equivalent hormonal treatment is the most like your own body. Before we take a look at what to do to make these symptoms go away, it is crucial that we first examine just how complex our bodies' hormonal processes are as well as how hormones are made and how they work.

Our bodies have been created to function in an environment of balance, where everything works together like a well-oiled machine. When the hormones within the body are balanced, health and well-being exist. Hormones are the chemical messengers within the body—they travel slowly within the bloodstream to tissues and organs to affect processes throughout the body, including:

- Growth and development
- Metabolism—how the body gets energy from foods
- Sexual function
- Reproduction
- Mood
- Brain function

As we previously discussed, hormones work slowly and they are very powerful. It takes only a tiny amount to cause big changes in cells or in the entire body. Too much or too little of a certain hormone can be serious.

As you can see by the list above, hormones are very important to the well-being of the body. As a matter of fact, physical health and emotional health are both intimately dependent on the body being balanced physically, spiritually, emotionally and mentally—all of which depend on hormone balance.

Certain hormones are produced by a group of glands and organs in the body called the endocrine system. The endocrine glands, including the pituitary gland, thyroid gland, pancreas, adrenal glands, ovaries and testicles are specialized glands that secrete their hormones directly into the bloodstream. All other glands including the salivary and breast, deliver their products by a tube called a duct. Whether the hormones are delivered directly into the bloodstream from the endocrine glands or substances via a duct, the body ensures that the hormones are properly delivered—at the right times and in the

"As a matter of fact, physical health and emotional health are both intimately dependent on the body being balanced physically, spiritually, emotionally and mentally—all of which depend on hormone balance."

right amounts—into the bloodstream.

Each one of the endocrine glands makes a specific hormone. Within the endocrine system, there are major glands that are present in both males and females, and there are glands that are only present in one or the other. The endocrine glands that are found in both sexes include the pituitary, pineal, thymus, thyroid, adrenal glands and pancreas. In addition to these hormone producing glands, men produce hormones in their testes and women produce hormones in their ovaries.

In the next chapter, we will discuss the endocrine system in depth to provide an extensive overview of each gland and the hormone it produces. You will need to understand this section so that you can know the questions to ask your physician when you are discussing hormonal imbalance with him.

Chapter 4

The Power of the Body's Endocrine System

"Hormones act as messengers to help regulate and coordinate activities throughout the body."
—The Merck Manual

Let's talk a little about the endocrine system and how it works within your body. What is the endocrine system and what are the glands and organs that comprise this system and what is the purpose of each hormone produced by each of the glands and organs?

Two systems control all physiologic processes in the human body:

- **The nervous system**, which exerts point-to-point control through nerves, similar to sending messages by conventional telephone. Nervous control is electrical in nature and fast.
- **The endocrine system,** which broadcasts its hormonal messages to essentially all cells by secretion into blood and

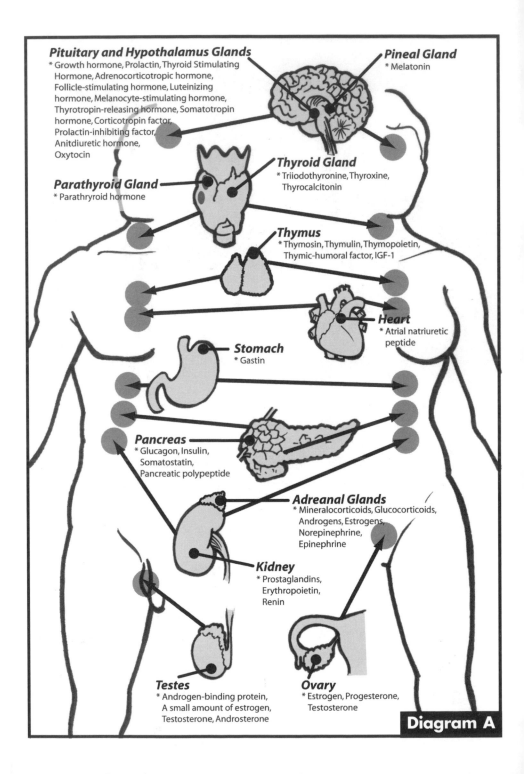

Pituitary and Hypothalamus Glands
* Growth hormone, Prolactin, Thyroid Stimulating
  Hormone, Adrenocorticotropic hormone,
  Follicle-stimulating hormone, Luteinizing
  hormone, Melanocyte-stimulating hormone,
  Thyrotropin-releasing hormone, Somatotropin
  hormone, Corticotropin factor,
  Prolactin-inhibiting factor,
  Anitdiuretic hormone,
  Oxytocin

Pineal Gland
* Melatonin

Parathyroid Gland
* Parathryroid hormone

Thyroid Gland
* Triiodothyronine, Thyroxine,
  Thyrocalcitonin

Thymus
* Thymosin, Thymulin, Thymopoietin,
  Thymic-humoral factor, IGF-1

Stomach
* Gastin

Heart
* Atrial natriuretic
  peptide

Pancreas
* Glucagon, Insulin,
  Somatostatin,
  Pancreatic polypeptide

Adreanal Glands
* Mineralocorticoids, Glucocorticoids,
  Androgens, Estrogens,
  Norepinephrine,
  Epinephrine

Kidney
* Prostaglandins,
  Erythropoietin,
  Renin

Testes
* Androgen-binding protein,
  A small amount of estrogen,
  Testosterone, Androsterone

Ovary
* Estrogen, Progesterone,
  Testosterone

Diagram A

extra-cellular fluid. Like a radio broadcast, it requires a receiver to get the message—in the case of endocrine messages, cells must bear a *receptor* for the hormone being broadcast in order to respond.

Communicating, Controlling, and Coordinating the Body's Work

Endocrinology is the study of chemical communication systems that provide the means to control a huge number of physiologic processes. Like other communication networks, the endocrine system contains transmitters, signals and receivers that are called, respectively, hormone producing cells, hormones and receptors.

The endocrine system is one of the many systems within the human body that work together to maintain health and balance. The responsibilities of the endocrine system include:

- Maintaining body energy levels
- Reproduction
- Growth and development
- Internal balance of body systems, called homeostasis
- Responses to surroundings, stress, and injury

The Pathophysiology of the Endocrine System

A particular cell is a target cell for a hormone if it contains functional receptors for that hormone, and cells which do not have such a receptor cannot be influenced directly by that hormone. Reception of a radio broadcast provides a good analogy. Everyone within range of a transmitter for National Public Radio is exposed to that signal. However, in order to be an NPR target and thus influenced directly by their broadcasts, you have to have a receiver tuned to that frequency. Hormone receptors are found either exposed on the surface of the cell or within the cell, depending on the type of hormone. In very basic terms, binding of hormone to receptor triggers a cascade of reactions within the cell that affects function.

How Does the Endocrine System Accomplish Its Responsibilities?

A network of glands and organs within the endocrine system produce, store, and secrete certain hormones (special chemicals that move into body fluid after they are made by one cell or a group of cells). Hormones cause an effect on other cells or tissues of the body.

The endocrine glands make the hormones that are used within our bodies. They produce the hormones and store them until needed. When the body sends out a call that it needs one of the hormones, the bloodstream carries them to the site. Now you can see that if the glands are not working properly and/or the bloodstream is not working properly, the system can fail. In addition to the glands and bloodstream, the receptors on the target cells must do their work, and there must be a system in place to control how hormones are produced and used. What a complicated system this is.

Things can and do go wrong within this system. Endocrine disorders happen when one or more of the systems we just described are not working. Sometimes there are not enough receptors, or binding sites for the hormones to direct the work that needs to be done. There may be a problem with the regulating of the hormones in the bloodstream, or something in the body is causing it not to regulate the hormone levels properly.

Glands are very small, yet powerful organs that are dispersed throughout the body. They are in control of releasing hormones.

Let's discuss the glands and organs that comprise the endocrine system so that you can get a better understanding of how this system works and certainly gain an appreciation of its importance within the body.

The Pituitary Gland—is the body's chief executive officer (CEO) or the "master gland." It has great influence on the other body organs. While its function is very complex, it is important for overall well-being.

It is a bean-sized gland that sits at the base of the brain just above the area where the nerves from the eyes meet. The pituitary gland is the command center regulating almost all hormones secreted from the endocrine glands. The endocrine glands secrete their hormones directly into the bloodstream and not through a duct like the glands that make sweat or saliva do. The pituitary gland is divided into two parts that sit one behind the other. The front half of the gland is called the anterior pituitary and regulates the production and the release of hormones from the thyroid gland, the adrenal gland, the ovaries, and the testicles. The hormones secreted from these glands control and regulate the release of hormones from all of the other endocrine glands except the pancreas.

Hormones secreted from the anterior pituitary include the very important:

1. **Follicle-stimulating hormone (FSH)**
   Exerts its control on the ovaries and testicles to regulate estrogen production in women and promotes sperm production in men.
2. **Luteinizing hormone (LH)**
   Regulates the production of estrogen in women and testosterone in men.
3. **Thyroid stimulating hormone (TSH)**
   Stimulates the thyroid gland to make thyroid hormones (T3 and T4), which, in turn, control (regulate) the body's metabolism, energy, growth and development, and nervous system activity.
4. **Adrenocorticotropic hormone (ACTH)**
   Stimulates production of cortisol by the adrenal glands. Cortisol, a so-called "stress hormone," is vital to survival. It helps maintain blood pressure and blood glucose levels.
5. **Growth hormone or GH**
   Stimulates growth in childhood and is important for maintaining a healthy body composition. In adults it is also important for maintaining muscle mass and bone mass. It can affect fat distribution in the body.

Hormones secreted from the posterior pituitary include:

1. Prolactin or PRL

Stimulates milk production from a woman's breasts after childbirth and can affect sex hormone levels from the ovaries in women and the testes in men.

2. Oxytocin

Causes milk letdown in nursing mothers and contractions during childbirth.

3. Antidiuretic hormone or ADH

Also called vasopressin, is stored in the back part of the pituitary gland and regulates water balance. If this hormone is not secreted properly, it can lead to problems of sodium (salt) and water balance and may also affect the kidneys.

Over- or under-production of pituitary hormones can cause the target glands (the glands affected by the pituitary hormones) to produce too many or too few hormones of their own.

To understand how each one of the endocrine hormones is controlled, it's important to know how the release of these hormones is regulated by the pituitary gland.

The regulation process is called the Feedback System—a very specific but delicate process. In Figure One, you will see a graphic depiction that shows the pituitary gland and how it works as the body's command center through a process called the Feedback System. The other glands send their hormones through the bloodstream. In the pituitary gland there are specific areas which control each gland. This means that each gland has a very specific site that controls its hormone production and release in the same way as a bank has a loan department and a trust department. An example of how this works can be seen in Figure One. The pituitary gland, through its blood supply, samples each hormone (estrogen, thyroid, etc.) that is in the specific area from which it is controlled. If the pituitary gland detects an

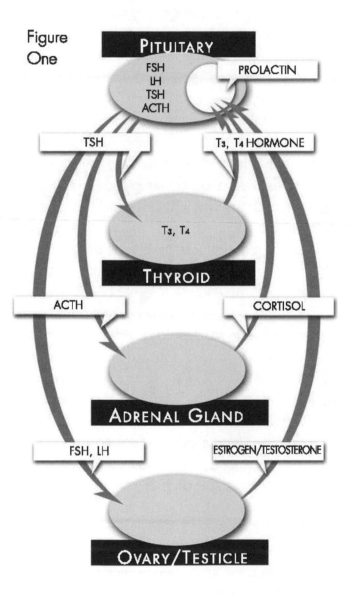

Figure One

abnormality in the production of any hormone by another gland, it sends a "regulatory hormone" to that gland and advises the gland to either make more hormone or less hormone, depending on the need.

A regulatory hormone is a hormone that by its action on certain cells within certain glands controls the production and release of those hormones from those specific glands. The majority of the regulatory hormones are produced by the pituitary gland at the base of the brain. The regulatory hormones affect the thyroid gland, the ovaries, the testicles, and the adrenal glands. In essence, your entire well-being is predicated on the body's ability to produce normal amounts of regulatory hormones. Without them, the thyroid, ovaries, testicles, and adrenal glands would cease to function properly and the human body would be plunged into disease.

Let's take the thyroid gland as an example. The thyroid hormone is brought to the pituitary gland where its level is determined in the thyroid area of the gland. If the thyroid gland isn't making enough hormone the pituitary gland determines how low the level of hormone is, then releases the proper amount of the regulatory hormone, thyroid stimulating hormone (TSH). The TSH then moves to the thyroid gland and tells the gland to make more hormone. The thyroid gland obeys and makes more hormone. Then, as the thyroid hormone level rises, the pituitary gland recognizes this information and begins to decrease the release of the regulatory hormone, in this case TSH. To simply describe the Feedback System, the pituitary gland finds a low hormone level and sends a messenger to that specific gland telling it to make more hormone. As the hormone levels rise, their information "feeds back" to the pituitary gland. The level of hormone in the blood is the information that feeds back to the pituitary, which then decides if the gland is overproducing or underproducing hormone. This process, known as the Feedback System or Feedback Mechanism, occurs rapidly. In the time it took to read the previous sentence, this process has taken place hundreds of times in your body. It continues every minute for twenty-four hours a day. The body needs steady levels of all hormones in the bloodstream at all times and functions optimally when the levels of all hormones are kept in a steady level flow.

The only method at this time that is able to deliver estrogen and testosterone in a steady continuous manner for a prolonged period of time (four to six months) is with the use of the pellet hormone delivery system (PHDS) equivalent hormone therapy.

Each of the regulatory hormones from the pituitary gland is gland specific; FSH (Follicle Stimulating Hormone), LH (Luteinizing Hormone), TSH (Thyroid Stimulating Hormone), ACTH (Adrenocorticotropic hormone), and Prolactin, which is the hormone from the posterior pituitary that is usually only secreted during pregnancy or when a woman is breast-feeding. (If prolactin is secreted in any significant amount other than in pregnancy or breast-feeding, a disease or adverse reaction to medication is present. High prolactin level can stop ovulation and estrogen production. One sign of an elevated prolactin is milk production from the nipple outside of pregnancy or breast-feeding.

Clearly, you can see from what you have just read that if the pituitary gland is malfunctioning, a considerable number of organs in the endocrine system can be affected. Pituitary tumors, cancerous and non-cancerous, can cause considerable upset in the human body. Diseases such as Sheehan's Syndrome, which occurs after the blood supply to the pituitary is stopped or suddenly reduced after delivery of a baby, can destroy the ability of the pituitary to produce regulatory hormones. This situation then produces serious health problems. I am continually amazed to find that so many physicians who do HRT for men and women still remain so hesitant to obtain blood levels of these regulatory hormones during routine evaluations or often at a patient's request.

The Thyroid Gland—Small But Powerful

The thyroid gland is a small organ within the endocrine system, weighing merely twenty grams, or less than an ounce, found in the neck beneath the Adam's apple. Despite its small size, it is one of the most important hormone-secreting organs in your body. The vital hormone secreted by the thyroid gland affects every cell in your body. Thyroid hormone therefore has an immense job maintaining the integrity and function of your entire body. And when this vital hormone is deficient, even in small amounts, it often results in a multitude of symptoms and conditions affecting every organ in your body.

The vital hormone secreted by the thyroid gland affects every cell in your body.

Some Common Misconceptions About the Thyroid

When speaking with patients at consults a lot of confusion exists about their thyroid. However, patients often come to me with a wealth of understanding and knowledge about estrogen and testosterone replacement and its importance to health and disease prevention. Patients fear a diagnosis about their thyroid believing that it may require surgery and "medication" for the rest of their lives. But thyroid hormone replacement is an equivalent strategy to estrogen and testosterone replacement.

Patients often do not realize that when a doctor diagnoses hypothyroidism, or a low functioning thyroid, that most of the time it involves simply replacing the hormone that the thyroid is failing to secrete. Also, patients have not been informed by their doctor that the "medication" that they receive for hypothyroidism is simply a hormone. In fact, it is a equivalent hormone. I have patients who have taken thyroid hormone replacement for decades and all along did not realize that it was a hormone. So, the bias towards taking a thyroid "medication" is created because many patients do not want to be reliant on taking some kind of pharmaceutical for the rest of their lives if they can avoid it. But thyroid hormone replacement offers the same clinical and health strategy as does estrogen and testosterone replacement therapy. This is disease prevention and improved quality of life through reduction of symptoms and optimization of energy and vitality.

How Does My Thyroid Help Me?

One of the important organs in the body that often undergoes changes before, during, and after menopause is the thyroid gland. At my clinic, approximately half of the new female patients that I see every day are already taking some kind of thyroid hormone replacement for hypothyroidism. In fact, epidemiological studies show that hypothyroidism is far more common in women, and especially women of menopausal age or with a family history of hypothyroidism. When underlying hypothyroidism already exists in a menopausal woman, the symptoms related to menopause become amplified. If a woman makes the decision to pursue estrogen PHDS therapy and testosterone PHDS therapy, it is important that we properly evaluate her thyroid function with a goal of gaining complete symptom relief and total body balance.

A few basic facts about hypothyroidism:

- Hypothyroidism affects twenty million Americans, or one in every ten people.
- Epidemiological surveys demonstrate hypothyroidism is up to eight times more common in women than men.
- Hypothyroidism runs in families, specifically among other females in the family such as a mother, aunt, grandmother, or sister.
- Surveys performed by the Thyroid Service of Harvard Medical School and the University of Colorado Health Sciences Center have estimated that by age fifty, one out of every ten to twelve women has some level of hypothyroidism. By age sixty, it is as common as one out of every five or six women.

The following list of symptoms is consistent with hypothyroidism. If you are suffering from any of these, speak with your family physician regarding treatment.

Early symptoms (you may notice these feelings in the early stages of hypothyroidism):

- Weakness
- Fatigue

- Cold intolerance
- Constipation
- Weight gain (unintentional)
- Depression
- Joint or muscle pain
- Thin, brittle fingernails
- Thin and brittle hair
- Paleness

Late symptoms (you may experience these problems in a later stage of hypothyroidism):

- Slow speech
- Dry flaky skin
- Thickening of the skin
- Puffy face, hands and feet
- Decreased taste and smell
- Thinning of eyebrows
- Hoarseness
- Abnormal menstrual periods

Additional symptoms that may be associated with this disease (If you notice any of these symptoms persisting, discuss the possibility of hypothyroidism with your physician):

- Overall swelling
- Muscle spasms (cramps)
- Muscle pain
- Muscle atrophy
- Uncoordinated movement
- Absent menstruation
- Joint stiffness
- Dry hair

- Hair loss
- Drowsiness
- Appetite loss
- Ankle, feet, and leg swelling
- Short stature
- Separated sutures
- Delayed formation or absence of teeth

Why Is There So Much Reported Hypothyroidism?

Hypothyroidism is often related, at some point in its course, to a stressor introduced into the endocrine system. And thyroid tissue is susceptible to stressors. Thyroid tissue is very delicate and is located in a relatively vulnerable position. Due to its extensive blood supply and the ability to trap nutrients for hormone synthesis, it is susceptible to many chemicals we encounter every day. The stressors I refer to can be defined as mental, emotional, spiritual, physical, or chemical. There is often a specific event or stressor that seems to mark the beginning of not feeling well. Patients will say, "Ever since I had my surgery (example only), I have never been the same."

"Common stressors patients may experience that are related to hypothyroidism:[34,39]

Chemical

- Lack of estrogen and testosterone that coincides with menopause and/or andropause
- Certain medications known to interfere with thyroid function (i.e. Lithium, Cordarone/amiodarone)
- Nutrient deficiencies such as iodine, selenium, or zinc
- Pollutants known to interfere with thyroid function (i.e., excess inorganic iodine, polychlorinated biphenyls [PCBs] from such sources as electrical equipment, DDT [banned insecticide] and many other pesticides, to name only a few).

Physical

- Direct trauma to the thyroid gland, i.e., surgeries around the neck
- Autoimmune processes that attack thyroid tissue (i.e., Hashimoto's thyroiditis)
- Whiplash injuries
- Excessive exercising
- Radiation exposure (i.e., medical or living or working close to a nuclear power plant)

Mental/Emotional/Spiritual

- Divorce
- Death in the family
- Loss of a job
- Promotion in your job leading to more responsibility
- Caring for an ailing family member"

How Does the Thyroid Work?

Thyroid Physiology—The Basics

Your thyroid gland is controlled by your brain just as all hormone secreting tissues are, just like the ovaries in women or testicles in men. A part of your brain called the hypothalamus sends a signal to your pituitary gland to secrete a hormone called Thyroid Stimulating Hormone (TSH). TSH is like an email message that is sent to the thyroid gland that simply says, "Make more thyroid hormone." When the thyroid is properly functioning, or actually home to answer the email, then the gland will secrete the thyroid hormone in response. Normally, when sufficient thyroid hormone is present in the body, the brain senses that the thyroid hormone levels are adequate and it becomes satisfied and stops sending down additional emails asking for more hormone.

- If the thyroid is sluggish, it cannot answer the email request to "make more thyroid hormone." The email messages start to pile up (in the mailbox of the thyroid) and TSH levels increase. This then leads to **hypothyroidism**, or low functioning thyroid.
- Sometimes, the thyroid gland dysfunctions and starts to overproduce thyroid hormone. The excessive levels of thyroid hormone in the blood are sensed by the pituitary gland. Additional emails from the pituitary, or TSH, are not sent out and consequently TSH levels become lower than normal. This is known as **hyperthyroidism**, or high functioning thyroid. This is much rarer than hypothyroidism.

The hypothalamus stimulates the pituitary gland to produce TSH, which then regulates the thyroid gland's production of thyroid hormone.

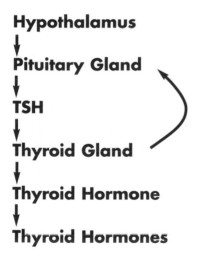

Hypothalamus

Pituitary Gland

TSH

Thyroid Gland

Thyroid Hormone

Thyroid Hormones

The main hormone that the thyroid produces is thyroxine or T4. It is also known as levothyroxine. It is called T4 because it has four iodine molecules surrounding a tyrosine molecule. This hormone is considered a prohormone—not the active hormone and does not directly affect cellular activity. Outside of the thyroid gland itself, T4 first needs to have one of the iodine molecules chopped off in a process called deiodination, yielding the active form of thyroid hormone called liothyronine or triiodothyronine, or simply T3.

- Levothyroxine (T4): The most abundantly produced thyroid hormone. A prohormone only and inactive.

- Liothyronine (T3): The active form of thyroid hormone that directly affects the body formed from T4. Liothyronine, or T3 affects a multitude of cells in the body. T3 helps your body:
  - Form bone and brain tissue in the fetus
  - Promote Growth Hormone production for normal growth
  - Lead to normal closure of the growth plates in bones
  - Regulate cell metabolism and energy
  - Increase core body temperature known as the Basal Metabolic Rate
  - Stimulate heart and lung tissue to function optimally
  - Control the function of the gastrointestinal system
  - Control the synthesis of serotonin, an important brain neurochemical
  - And much more

How Do I Know If I Have a Thyroid Disorder?

Here are some of the common symptoms related to hypothyroidism. Remember, thyroid hormone is responsible for the proper function of every cell in your body, so the list of symptoms and conditions ranges from head to toe, inside and out.(2,7)

- Extreme fatigue
- Weight gain despite exercise and diet
- Thinning hair
- Poor appetite
- Slow thinking
- Choking sensation

- Dry and course skin
- Insensitive to the cold
- Constipation and/or diarrhea
- Depression and anxiety
- Shortness of breath
- Swelling around/above the eyes
- Swollen face
- Brittle nails with heavy ridges

There are also many medical conditions that are related to hypothyroidism. Infertility, menstrual disturbances, psychiatric conditions, fibromyalgia, autoimmune diseases such as rheumatoid arthritis and lupus, Raynaud's phenomena, and insulin-dependent diabetes are all associated with hypothyroidism. Having one of these conditions increases your risk for being or becoming hypothyroid.[34,39]

The more common ones that I see on a daily basis are:

- Hypotension: low blood pressure, normally seen in the beginning stages of hypothyroidism (i.e., ninety/sixty or less is considered low)
- Hypertension: high blood pressure, normally seen in the later stages of hypothyroidism (greater than one hundred forty/ninety consistently)
- Gastroesophageal reflux disease (GERD): chronic symptoms or mucosal damage produced by the abnormal reflux of gastric contents into the esophagus
- Irritable Bowel Syndrome (IBS): cramping, abdominal pain, bloating, constipation, and diarrhea
- Hyperlipidemia: elevated cholesterol and other blood lipids (fats) such as triglycerides and LDL or 'bad cholesterol'

It's difficult to say just how many hypothyroid patients I see who also have these common conditions and depend on additional medications for them. These conditions are representative of the ones that would largely be managed without the need for additional medications if they were properly diagnosed as patients with hypothyroidism and/or treated with an appropriate dose of thyroid hormone. This is especially true of patients with high cholesterol levels. If a patient is given a proper dose of thyroid hormone, cholesterol levels will almost invariably come down.

Testing Thyroid Function
Blood Tests

There are several blood tests that can be performed to accurately assess thyroid function. If your physician is attempting to determine your thyroid status, the blood test panel should consist of the following.[34,39]

TSH: Thyroid Stimulating Hormone

The TSH level blood test is one of the basic tests that are run to determine thyroid function. It was first designed by researchers as a test for "disease potential." In other words, it is a limited test that only suggests dysfunction of the thyroid gland and its related hormones. When the brain senses low levels of thyroid hormone in the blood circulation, TSH is secreted from the pituitary in the brain to "stimulate" or signal the thyroid gland to produce thyroid hormone for the body. The thyroid gland in turn secretes thyroid hormone and this hormone finally signals the brain to stop secreting more TSH, in a negative feedback loop.

The normal range: in 2003 the American Association of Clinical Endocrinologists changed the recommendations for the normal range of TSH to (zero point three to three point zero). However, not all laboratories use this new range. Some of the laboratories use ranges that go up as high as six. *The higher the TSH value goes, the greater low functioning (hypothyroid) the thyroid may be.* If the value of TSH is below zero point three, it may imply high functioning (hyperthyroidism) of the thyroid gland. I use a range of (zero point three to two point zero) based on a large twenty-year English community study that demonstrated TSH ranges in individuals over two point zero indicated an increased risk of hypothyroidism.[45]

"Fine Tuning" Doses of Thyroid Hormone and TSH Suppression

One of the most glaring problems that I have observed in patients diagnosed with hypothyroidism has been the under treatment of thyroid hormone for their hypothyroidism. Despite being on thyroid hormone, sometimes for many years, they still suffer from the classic symptoms of hypothyroidism that brought them to their physician for their initial diagnosis. They also suffer from many related hypothyroid diseases that developed over the years while on inadequate doses of thyroid hormone. Their thyroid hormone dose has been limited based on the TSH (Thyroid Stimulating Hormone) blood test. This test, as explained before, is designed to screen for disease potential for hypothyroidism or hyperthyroidism (overactive thyroid). Many doctors use the test to keep the dose in the "correct" range, and even the interpretation of what range is correct will vary from physician to physician. This is called "fine tuning" the thyroid dose to the TSH. Their rationale for this is that if the TSH gets too low from a particular dose of thyroid hormone, then that dose is too high.

Many endocrinologists and other physicians incorrectly believe that if the TSH is "suppressed" or too low from a specific thyroid hormone dose then it will lead to problems with your heart and increase your risk for osteoporosis. This has never been proven scientifically and there is a wealth of recent scientific data to show that these types of symptom-relieving doses do not cause any problems with your heart or your bones.[33,36,37,38,40,41,42,43]

Total T4 or T4 (RIA)

Total T4 is a direct measurement of thyroxine being secreted from the thyroid. Thyroxine is the main thyroid hormone that is secreted from the thyroid, but it has minimal activity and minimal effect on the function of cells. In hypothyroidism, the total T4 value is at the low or low end of normal. In hyperthyroidism, the value is increased.

Total T3

The T3 blood test is a direct measurement of T3 level, or thyronine, circulating in the blood. Most of the T3 found in the blood is created in the body when T4 is converted in active T3. Only small amounts of T3 are secreted from the thyroid. This measurement is important because T3 is the only active form of thyroid hormone that positively affects body cells.

Free T4

The T4 blood test measures the available unbound amount of T4 in the blood. Some of the T4 in the blood is bound by a protein called thyroid binding globulin (TBG). Free T4 is directly available to the cells to be converted into active T3. In hypothyroidism, the free T4 value is decreased. In hyperthyroidism, the value is often increased.

Free T3

The Free T3 blood test is very similar to free T4 blood test and functions in the same way. However, this test is more useful in the diagnosis of hyperthyroidism.

Anti-TPO and Anti-Tg Antibodies

The Anti-TPO (thyroid peroxidase) and the Anti-Tg antibodies blood tests measure the amount of antibodies to thyroid tissue that are present in the body. When present in high amounts, these antibodies demonstrate that a possible autoimmune process is occurring in the body leading to Hashimoto's thyroiditis—the most common form of thyroiditis. Classified as an autoimmune disorder, Hashimoto's thyroiditis causes an autoimmune reaction with antibodies attacking the thyroid gland. The antibodies are proteins that are produced by the body's immune system that are produced in high amounts for unclear reasons. These antibodies attack and destroy thyroid tissue over time. High levels of anti-TPO and anti-Tg antibodies therefore increase the risk of hypothyroidism.

Additional Tests

Blood tests have two inherent weaknesses when it comes to thyroid hormone diagnosis and treatment. First of all, they do not exclusively reflect whether or not a patient is hypothyroid or hyperthyroid. And secondly, the use of thyroid hormone tests to clinically determine a patient's particular dose of thyroid hormone is not always accurate. There are additional tests that assist both the diagnosis and the individualized course of treatment for hypothyroidism or hyperthyroidism.

Basal Metabolic Rate (BMR) Analysis

The BMR is the rate at which the body uses energy while at rest. This test uses a machine that measures the specific metabolism or oxygen consumption of the entire body that indicates the amount of energy a body is using. Since thyroid hormone affects metabolism within all cells of the body, this test proves to be one of the best indirect measurements of overall metabolism and therefore thyroid hormone function.

Basal Body Temperature (BBT)

The BBT is relatively reliable in determining the basal metabolic rate of an individual. It is not as accurate as the extensive machines used to measure basal metabolic rate but is a simple and inexpensive test that employs an ordinary glass thermometer to take the temperature when the patient is truly resting when they first wake in the morning. If thyroid hormone function is low, the basal metabolic rate is low, and therefore the basal body temperature is *often* low. The opposite is *often* true in hyperthyroidism (high thyroid function). The basal body temperature should be at least ninety-seven point eight degrees Fahrenheit and no higher than ninety-eight point two degrees Fahrenheit. It is not uncommon for hypothyroid patients to start out with a basal body temperature as low as ninety-five degrees Fahrenheit. Patients often believe that the thermometer is broken when they discover how low the value can actually be. But through the course of treatment, often the temperature increases along with their symptomatic improvement.

I have found the BBT test to be useful from a clinical standpoint in both the diagnosis and especially the treatment of hypothyroidism. It is important to note that it is not a perfect test and is not always accurate. I use it in conjunction with proper clinical judgment and the other laboratory and complimentary tests.

Achilles Reflex Testing

In general, all body reflexes are affected by thyroid function. In hypothyroidism, when thyroid function is low, the body reflexes are slow. In hyperthyroidism, when thyroid function is excessive, then the body reflexes are fast. The Achilles tendon is located just above the heel bone and is easily accessed by the clinician.

The Achilles reflex test is another simple clinical test that proves to be generally consistent in supporting the diagnosis of a thyroid disorder and determining if treatment is effective. It is important to note that this test can be affected by other factors such as certain medications, nutrient deficiencies, and neurological problems. Just as any clinical or laboratory test, it is only a tool and must be used in conjunction with sound clinical judgment.

Nutrition for the Thyroid

There are many nutrients that benefit thyroid gland function. The most important ones include iodine, selenium, and zinc, which are needed for the synthesis and function of the thyroid gland and its hormones. To ensure healthy thyroid function in general, the diet should contain natural sources of selenium, zinc and iodine including various sea foods such as shrimp and lobster, kelp sources found in many Japanese foods such as sushi, and various raw nuts such as Brazil nuts. Replacing your table salt used for flavoring and cooking with Celtic sea salt is an effective and extremely tasty way to increase these and other minerals in the diet. This form of salt will not increase your blood pressure.

Thyroid Hormone Replacement Options

If your healthcare provider has determined that you present clinically with hypothyroidism, a likely course of action will be to offer thyroid hormone replacement therapy. There are many options you should carefully explore both through your own research and with your doctor. (Please see the back of this book for a list of Web sites you can access to gain more information.)

Levothyroxine or T4:

Common manufactured brands for Levothyroxine or T4 are Synthroid and Levoxyl. This is the typical form of treatment employed by endocrinologists and other practitioners. It is technically a equivalent hormone, but is also synthetic hormone.

Triiodothyronine, Liothyronine or T3

The most popular brand of Triiodothyronine/Liothyronine or T3 in the United States is Cytomel. This particular form of thyroid hormone is not often prescribed by a typical endocrinologist or family practice physician. Cytomel is equivalent and synthetically produced.

Compounded T4 (Levothyroxine) and T3 (Triiodothyronine) Combinations

A compounding pharmacist can provide a combination of T4 and T3 in an individualized dose that is appropriate for a patient but may not be available in a manufactured brand name of thyroid hormone. The hormones compounding pharmacists are equivalent hormones manufactured by the human body.

Armour Thyroid

This is one of the oldest forms of thyroid hormone treatment and is highly cost effective. It is a USP (United States Pharmacopoeia) standardized form of porcine (pig) thyroid tissue that is a natural thyroid hormone replacement and it is not synthetic. It is equivalent in structure.

Nature-Throid

This particular form of glandular thyroid hormone is very similar to Armour thyroid because it also uses USP porcine sources for its products. However, it far more hypoallergenic, meaning a patient is less likely to develop allergic responses to the product. The principal difference from Armour is that Nature–Throid does not contain corn starch as a binder like Armour, and this lowers the allergic response for many patients who have various food allergies. The product is also free from dyes and other preservatives that are present in Armour.

The Adrenal Glands

The Adrenal glands are two glands, each is actually two endocrine organs, that work together and sit like hats above each kidney. Even though there is one adrenal gland on each side of the body, they work as one gland. The adrenal glands have an outer covering resembling the peel of an orange, called the adrenal cortex. This peel-like layer produces glucocorticoids (such as cortisol)—very important in helping the body to control blood sugar, increase the burning of protein and fat, and respond to stressors like fever, major illness, and injury. The mineral corticoids (such as aldosterone) control blood volume and help to regulate blood pressure by acting on the kidneys to help them hold onto enough sodium and water. The adrenal cortex also produces some sex hormones, which are important for some secondary sex characteristics in both men and women.

The production and the release of our internally manufactured cortisone (called cortisol) are regulated by the pituitary hormone, adrenocorticotropic hormone (ACTH). This is controlled by another Feedback System. (See Figure One. The pituitary gland sends the messenger hormone, ACTH, which tells the adrenal glands when the body is under stress so that they can make cortisol. The adrenal glands respond by making and releasing cortisol. When enough hormones are sent back to the pituitary gland through the bloodstream, the area in the pituitary that produces the messenger hormone ACTH recognizes the body has enough of the hormone, cortisol, and turns off the production of ACTH when enough hormone has been made.

When diseases or tumors affect the adrenal glands, life-threatening conditions arise. Diseases that affect or destroy the adrenal glands can adversely affect our immune system, blood pressure, heart function, weight control, and muscles. The spongy middle of the adrenal gland, which can be compared to the pulp of an orange, is called the medulla. This spongy middle produces adrenaline, which is what speeds up our heart rate, increases our blood pressure, and gets us ready to deal with stress. When we humans are under stress and we get sweaty and our hearts race, it is because of the amount of adrenaline the adrenal gland makes. The more adrenaline released, the more our hearts race and the more we feel sweaty. If you ever get a shot of adrenaline to treat the effects of an allergy reaction or an attack of asthma you rapidly find out your heart speeds up significantly, making you shake, tremble and sweat.

The adrenal glands can also produce small amounts of estrogen and testosterone which can be overproduced in times of stress, or in response to disease or tumors. It is not unusual for women to develop irregular periods, acne, and fluid retention as a result of stress or disease causing the adrenal glands to overproduce estrogen, testosterone and weaker forms of male-like hormones.

The Pancreas

The pancreas is a large gland in the digestive and endocrine systems, located behind the stomach, that is both exocrine (secreting pancreatic juice containing digestive enzymes) and endocrine (producing several important hormones, including insulin, glucagons, and somatostatin). Blood sugar regulation and production of digestive enzymes are the main functions of the pancreas. The pancreas sits to the right of the stomach, close to the gallbladder. Its proximity to the gallbladder is why diseases of the gallbladder can cause the pancreas to become inflamed. The pancreas is a soft gland that has small groups of cells called the Islets of Langerhans that produce the hormone insulin. Insulin secretion is regulated by the "feedback" of the body's blood sugar to these groups of cells.

When blood sugar rises, these cells produce insulin to drive the sugar into the body's cells to be utilized as fuel. When the body can no longer produce adequate insulin, the disease, diabetes, develops. The severity of the diabetes depends on how much insulin the body can produce. The less insulin produced in response to an increase in blood sugar, the more severe the diabetes becomes. Recent development of effective drugs to help diabetes sufferers who still have the ability to produce some insulin has been a great step forward in therapy. These individuals usually have developed diabetes as adults (Adult Onset Diabetes) or Type II. The more serious form of the disease is called Insulin Dependent Diabetes (IDD) or Type I. Patients with IDD must give themselves multiple injections of insulin as a daily routine to regulate their blood sugar. Researchers have determined that regulation of the body's blood sugar is best achieved with multiple doses of insulin. There is currently ongoing research in insulin therapy to create an insulin product that exhibits a steady secretion of insulin, or a recreation of what the body normally produces. Another important development is the development of human insulin. The use of this insulin by diabetics has eliminated adverse allergies that are often associated with the reactions to pig and horse insulin, which contained abnormal proteins which caused adverse reactions frequently. (Horse estrogen has the same problems.)

I hope that by now you are beginning to see a common thread developing through this discussion, not only related to the pancreas but to hormones in general. The common thread equivalent —exactly what the body produces—is the secret ingredient in medicine. Side effects are diminished or eliminated when a therapy, prescribed by doctors, uses precisely the same thing that is produced by the body naturally to supplement the body's own functions versus a process of imitation.

The pancreas produces the endocrine hormone insulin and has its own internal control or feedback mechanism. The groups of cells that produce insulin, which keeps the blood sugar normal, are called the Islets of Langerhans. These groups of cells produce insulin in response to the level of sugar present in the blood. The pituitary gland doesn't function in this process. The Islets control themselves. Historically, if insulin was needed, it was obtained from pigs and horses. It was found that these forms of insulin caused significant problems to patients who experienced adverse reactions. This was rectified when human insulin was developed. In addition, better control of the blood sugar has been realized by the use of multiple injections, because the blood sugar level stays much more consistently within the normal range. In fact, this prompted the development of a machine called the insulin pump which allows a steady stream of insulin to be continuously administered. The insulin pump releases biologically equivalent hormone in a low-dose steady stream and has the capability to give more when needed. This is the perfect model for replacing all endocrine hormones.

The Ovary

The ovary is an egg-producing reproductive organ present in females that is often found in pairs as part of the female reproductive system. Ovaries in females are similar to what testes are in males. The two ovaries, one on each side of a woman's body, are located next to the uterus. The two ovaries have cells that produce estrogen, progesterone and testosterone. The production and release of these hormones is controlled by a feedback mechanism involving the pituitary gland's production of Follicle Stimulating Hormone (FSH) and Luteinizing Hormone (LH), the two hormones that control the production and release of estrogen and progesterone during a menstrual cycle. (See Figure One.)

The pituitary hormones FSH and LH also control the process of ovulation (egg development and release). In addition, the ovaries have certain cells that produce only testosterone. With the tremendous impact on women of estrogen, progesterone, and testosterone deficiency, a separate chapter will be devoted to this alone including treatment with the PHDS of equivalent hormone replacement.

The Testicle

The testicle is the male reproductive gland that is usually found in pairs in most men. The testicles are contained within an extension of the abdomen called the scrotum. In men the testicles are responsible for testosterone hormone production and sperm production as well. Like the ovary, the testicles are controlled by the pituitary gland's production of FSH and LH through the feedback mechanism. See Figure One. Unlike the ovary, the testicle only produces one hormone, testosterone, when functioning normally. Men can produce small amounts of estrogen, but it's not made by any cell in the testicle but rather by the transformation of testosterone into the hormone estrogen by an enzyme. I will explain how this all happens in subsequent chapters.

CASE STUDIES

*Ann, a fifty-four-year-old woman, presented to me with a history of repeated complaints to her doctor of severe hot flashes and insomnia. She felt like her head was going to "blow off." Her physician had given her oral estrogen at age fifty-two and was reluctant to check her hormone levels. When the physician did test Ann's blood levels, it was only her estrogen level that was checked. It was found to be normal. The physician told Ann that there was nothing wrong with her estrogen and that she just needed to relax more. When Ann came to see me, I ordered a full hormone panel blood test, which demonstrated a normal estrogen, but her FSH level was very very high, indicating that her estrogen level was insufficient for her particular physiology. This was the cause of her continual hot flashes. The peaks and valleys being delivered by her oral estrogen were not delivering enough hormone. She was also very deficient in testosterone, which compounded the problem. After treatment with a course of estrogen and testosterone through the PHDS, her FSH level fell below twenty and her testosterone level rose to the normal range, functional levels, and her symptoms disappeared completely. As Ann so well put it, **"I haven't felt this good in years."**

William, a forty-five-year-old engineer, presented to me with a history of loss of muscle mass, a low libido, feelings of poor energy, and a lack of mental clarity. He related that he could no longer exercise to the level he once did and had uncontrolled weight gain in spite of diet and regular exercise. His blood work showed a low testosterone level, an elevated estrogen level, high LH level and high FSH level. He was treated with testosterone pellets by way of the PHDS and a medication to stop his estrogen production. In his own words, he told me, **"I've got normal energy; I can exercise normally again and most importantly I can think clearly."** Unfortunately, his problems were written off by his other physicians due to stress and "you're to young" to have hormone problems.

Hormones — The Vital Link

The endocrine system functions well in older people, despite changes that happen as we age. The Hormone Foundation notes that some of these changes happen because of normal cell aging and may alter the following:

- Hormone production and secretion
- Hormone metabolism
- Hormone levels circulating in the bloodstream
- Biological activities within the body
- Target cell or target tissue response to hormones
- Rhythms in the body, such as menstrual cycle

Human hormones are substances our bodies produce to regulate and stimulate many organ systems. Without a balance in the levels of hormones within our bodies, they are swept into a state of chaos and disease. Hormones keep us on a normal balanced path which helps us maintain wellness and fight off illness. Often physicians forget how important proper hormone balance is to the maintenance of overall well-being. This often leads to patients not being evaluated completely and being told or made to feel that what they are experiencing is "all in your head." In truth, many of the feelings of illness you might be feeling can be hormone-based, and the imbalance of hormones is not imaginary.

Hopefully, the previous discussion on control of hormone production and release by means of the Feedback System (see Figure One) has been sufficient to give you at least a clearer understanding of how the endocrine glands (pituitary, thyroid, pancreas, adrenals, ovaries and testicles) work.

Estrogen and Progesterone

"Hormones keep us on a normal balanced path which helps us maintain wellness and fight off illness."

Figure Two demonstrates in a simple way how our bodies make the hormones—estrogen and progesterone. As you can see everything starts with the cholesterol molecule. If one's diet is inadequate, it can affect the hormones' output in the body. Human hormones are substances our bodies produce to regulate, stimulate, and affect many organ systems. Without these, many of the things we do every day would be impossible. Hormones keep us on a normal, balanced path that will lead us to total wellness. When our bodies' natural processes are interrupted, we are placed in an unbalanced, diseased state where we are in a physical, mental, and emotional state termed an illness. How often have you or someone you know been told, "It's all in your head?" In truth, many of the things we see or experience as feeling ill are hormone based, and the imbalance of hormones produced in our bodies caused these problems. They are not imaginary!

Estrogen

The body makes three different estrogens: estrone, estradiol and estriol. The primary estrogen found in a woman is estradiol. In fact, it is produced in amounts twice as great as the levels of estrone in the blood. This ratio of estradiol to estrone normally is two to one. If a woman's body is to function normally, it has to maintain a normal ratio. If the ratio is changed, it would cause too much estrone to be made, and this estrogen is a very strong breast stimulator. One reason women complain of breast tenderness while on oral estrogens is because all oral estrogens do not keep the normal ratio of estradiol to estrone at two to one. In fact the ratio seen with Premarin™ and all tablets containing conjugated estrogens is a complete reversal of this ratio to

Figure Two

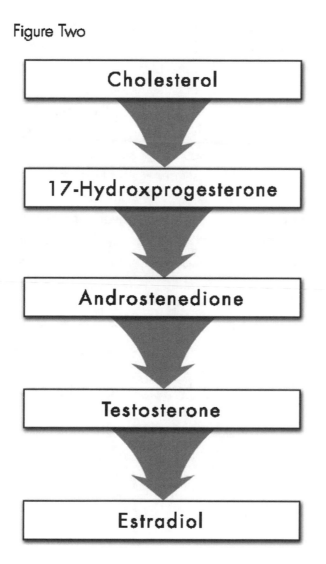

one to two. The oral estradiol (i.c., Estrace™) tablets usually make the normal ratio of two to one change to one to one. This identical ratio is also seen with the estradiol used in all the estrogen patches. The only form of estrogen therapy that reproduces the normal ratio of estrogens in the body is the type used in the PHDS (estradiol pellets). Dr. Thom's articles published in 1980 and 1981 in the British Journal of Medicine and British Journal of OB/GYN demonstrated this very elegantly.

Estriol has been touted as an estrogen that does not cause breast cancer. The evidence for this is faulty. The amount of estriol used in these studies was so low that the estrogen level in the blood would be very low. If enough estriol is given to produce a relief of symptoms of the menopause such as vaginal dryness and changing of hot flashes, the dosage would be two to four times the amount used in these studies. In fact any estrogen given in doses that equal the doses used in these studies would also show no increase in the incidence of breast cancer. This leads to only one conclusion. Give women the estrogen the body uses commonly, estradiol. Furthermore, recreate the normal ratio of estradiol to the other estrogens, two to one. And remember, the only form of estrogen replacement therapy that can do all of this is biologically equivalent PHDS therapy and the use of estradiol pellets.

R. D. Gambrell, Jr., MD, wrote a critical review of the findings of the Women's Health Initiative (WHI) Reports in 2004 in which he discussed in detail estrogen-only therapy. I am going to provide you with his insight into this report because it is very important that you completely understand the importance of estrogen therapy at specific times during your life. As Dr. Gambrell stated in this report, "There is little controversy that hormone therapy (HT) has a beneficial impact on postmenopausal quality of life, but the WHI did not reflect this. This is because the WHI results do not apply to the majority of HT users. Postmenopausal women must continue estrogen therapy (ET) in adequate dosages for many years to achieve the maximum benefits. The lowest effective dosage for the shortest period of time is invalid, as the benefits of long-term HT far exceed the risks—the WHI notwithstanding."

The benefits of estrogen/estrogen/progestogen therapy, as summarized by Dr. Gambrell, are:

- Relief of vasomotor symptoms
  - Hot flashes and night sweats
- Prevention of urogenital atrophy
  - Fifteen percent of premenopausal women, ten percent to forty percent of postmenopausal women, and ten percent to twenty-five percent of

women receiving systemic hormone therapy experience urogenital atrophy. The most common symptoms are dryness, burning, pruritus, irritation, and dyspareunia. Estrogen loss, drugs, and chemical sensitivities are causes. Estrogen or hormone replacement therapy (ERT-HRT) is the treatment of choice in postmenopausal women. Dosages prescribed for menopause symptoms or to prevent osteoporosis (and, potentially, other conditions) can restore the vagina to premenopausal physiology and relieve symptoms."[47]

- Alleviation of psychogenic manifestations
  - Psychologic symptoms can include anxiety, tension, depression, insomnia, palpitations, headaches and other psychosomatic complaints.
- Improved quality of life
- Prevention of osteoporosis
  - Osteoporosis affects twenty-five million older Americans; ninety percent of those affected are postmenopausal women. Approximately twenty-five percent of white women over sixty years of age have spinal compression fractures. These fractures are present in fifty percent of women by age seventy-five. Of all hip fractures, eighty percent are associated with osteoporosis, and thirty-four percent of elderly patients with hip fracture die within six months.[48]
- Prevention of cardiovascular disease
  - Myocardial infarction (MI) rarely occurs in premenopausal women. Several recent studies have suggested that estrogens may exert a protective effect against cardiovascular disease, especially when low dosages of natural estrogens sufficient to relieve menopausal symptoms are used.[49]
- Prevention of Alzheimer's disease
  - Alzheimer's disease (AD) involves the parts of the brain that control thought, memory, and language.
- Reduction in macular degeneration
  - Use of postmenopausal estrogen therapy appears to reduce the odds of advanced macular degeneration among post-

menopausal women who have macular degeneration. Women who had used postmenopausal estrogen therapy have fifty-four percent lower odds of advanced macular degeneration compared with nonusers.[50]

- Reduction in cataracts
  - According to the *Aging Eye*, published by the University of Illinois, longer duration of reproductive period, i.e., longer exposure to endogenous estrogen and/or use of estrogen replacement after menopause, may delay or reduce the severity of cortical and nuclear lens opacities in women.

Testosterone

Both men and women produce testosterone (See Figure Two.) Figure two gives a simple diagram of how testosterone is made. Men produce over ninety-nine percent of their testosterone in certain cells of the testicle and one percent from the adrenal gland. Women produce testosterone primarily from their ovaries and a tiny amount from the adrenal glands.

Postmenopausal women continue to produce testosterone from their ovaries even after estrogen production has stopped. Without the proper levels of testosterone, men and women experience loss of mental focus and concentration. The lack of testosterone also produces muscle loss, decreased strength, fatigue, poor response to exercise, loss of libido (sex drive and arousal), and worsened menopausal symptoms in women. Anxiety and irritability are increased in both men and women suffering from lack of testosterone. If men and women suffer when they are testosterone deficient, how should this be treated? The best option is natural biologically equivalent testosterone. Synthetic and chemically treated testosterone can cause serious problems such as facial hair, baldness, acne, liver problems and prostate problems.

Biologically equivalent testosterone is least likely to cause problems, especially when used in pellet form. The injection of synthetic testosterone causes the "roller coaster" effect just like estrogen injection. (The "roller coaster" effect is seen in the blood levels when bio-equivalent synthetic replicas pills, patches, or creams are used. The up and down swings of hormones are produced as a result of the length of the life cycle of each form of hormone therapy. The shorter the life of the hormone, the faster the rise and decline of the hormone levels in the blood.) Oral forms of testosterone, unless they are equivalent, can cause liver problems. To be complete, testosterone gels and creams are available, but they have to be applied many times daily to try and reproduce normal blood levels, which they don't.

The only form of equivalent testosterone that recreates the natural blood levels the body needs over an extended period (three to six months) is pellet therapy. To summarize, the only form of testosterone therapy that is safe and effective is the type of equivalent testosterone pellets used in PHDS therapy. The last aspect to be addressed is how PHDS testosterone therapy benefits men and women.

Other forms of testosterone therapy have major drawbacks—patches, creams, tablets, and injections—all of which produce a pronounced roller coaster effect. Furthermore, they enhance the production of a protein called SHBG (sex hormone binding globulin) into the blood that attaches itself to testosterone and renders it useless. PHDS hormones do not produce any of these negative effects.

Following initiation of pellet testosterone therapy, both sexes can expect increased sexual arousal, increased libido, improved mental acuity, improved mental focus and concentration, improved muscle tone, less fatigue, more energy, and improved bone density. Testosterone is a great bone builder and lack of it leads to the development of osteoporosis. The use of PHDS gives the body the doses needed over a long period of time that allow for improved bone production.

What is a normal testosterone level for women? In many of my clinics, women are often presenting with testosterone levels deemed to be normal by other physicians. They are often told their lack of energy and sex drive, loss of strength and muscle mass are due to normal aging. Often, they relate situations to me where they were told, "just live with it" or, "have an affair" to recharge their sex lives.

As you can well imagine, I was horrified to hear that a physician would say such things to a patient. Since the most commonly used tests for assessing testosterone levels are unreliable below three hundred[15] the actual normal testosterone range for women is erroneous. Therefore the "normal range" for testosterone needs to be reestablished because women are constantly being told they are normal, when they are actually deficient. For a woman to be normal using the present form of testing, she would need total testosterone levels of somewhere between eighty and one hundred fifty continuously.

When treatment is considered to establish normal testosterone levels, one must consider the PHDS for therapy because this type of hormone delivery will provide consistently normal levels. Other forms of delivery such as creams, provide very high (four hundred and greater) levels of testosterone within one to two hours. This then plunges rapidly as the hormone is absorbed. Peaks and valleys are abnormal in the human body. When I am designing a therapy for my patients, I try to establish a plateau range of total testosterone of eighty to one hundred fifty as my goal.

Men on the other hand, need their total testosterone to be in the range of what their bodies produced when they were in their thirties—seven hundred to eleven hundred. The free testosterone needs to be above the middle range of normal for either sex. As an example, the range for free testosterone is ten to forty with the midpoint being twenty-five. Deduct the difference between ten and forty, which is thirty, and divide it by two to get the midpoint (ten plus fifteen equals twenty-five). Use this formula to see if the value is in the "real" normal range.

The signs and symptoms of endocrine disorders (hormonal imbalance) affect many of the systems within the body. These signs and symptoms are often difficult to detect and may be incorrectly linked to other causes, such as normal hormonal changes or other medical disorders.

Because the aging process affects nearly every gland within the body, there is impaired secretion of some hypothalamic hormones or impaired pituitary response. The pituitary gland can become smaller and more fibrous and may not work as well. Aging can also affect a woman's ovaries: menopause. The ovaries stop responding to FSH and LH from the anterior pituitary. Ovarian production of estrogen and progesterone slows down and eventually stops.

Chapter 5

Gauging Your Body's Proper Balance through Appropriate Laboratory Testing

"What I dream of is an art of balance."
—Henri Matisse

Hormone balance cannot be achieved by guesswork or with inefficient information about any hormone replacement therapy. It is critical that your doctor order the correct laboratory work and understand what the results indicate—which too often is not the case.

Errors in diagnosis and/or treatment are often the results of inappropriate laboratory testing; incorrect laboratory work, or misinterpretation of the results of the completed laboratory testing. Therefore, it is in your best interest to find a healthcare provider who uses a scientific approach to hormone therapy and designs your personal therapy based on scientific evidence. This means that a healthcare provider who orders the appropriate laboratory workup from the very beginning will be more apt to make the correct diagnosis for you and, more importantly, will recheck the laboratory work again after therapy begins to assess the success of the therapy. If he finds that your therapy is not working as well as it should, he will then have the scientific basis to alter the therapeutic approach to achieve a more positive outcome.

So many times, patients have presented to me with copies of laboratory results indicating normal hormone levels, but there is no measurement of the corresponding regulatory hormone included in these results. When these patients were re-evaluated by me and the appropriate laboratory tests ordered, nearly all of them showed blood work results that indicated a need for hormone therapy, or the results showed that their present therapy was ineffective. These types of situations are ongoing occurrences in my practice. In many of these cases, the patients told me that their complaints to their healthcare providers went unheeded or ignored and this caused them to experience additional anxiety and often bouts of depression. A patient whose original laboratory work indicated normal hormone levels had no idea that her original healthcare provider had not measured the regulatory hormone. She was done a great disservice by that healthcare provider. The patient felt something was wrong, but couldn't put her finger on exactly what it was. When she asked her healthcare provider about this feeling, she was told that everything was normal. She interpreted this response to mean, "It's all in your head." Patients with similar experiences can't help but feel frustrated and helpless.

For so long we physicians have not been taught to check or recheck estrogen or FSH laboratory test values. More often than not, we have been taught to use the "I feel okay" test. If the patient complains of feeling miserable and then "feels okay" after a pill is given, then the physician is led to believe that he/she has done a "good job." In reality, we have only applied a Band-aid and not cured the problem. Why is this so often the standard of care? The only answer I can provide is just plain ignorance.

Historically, estrogen therapy has been practiced by physicians as if hormone pills are candy. Give a patient the green pill, red pill or how about the yellow pill until they say they are feeling better. Job done!

Where is the laboratory evidence that demonstrates whether that patient is normal again before and after a hormone is given? For all other types of illnesses, doesn't a thorough physician properly check all appropriate laboratory tests before and after all other types of therapy have been decided upon? Isn't he very careful to review every possible blood test before deciding on a medication to prescribe? And, doesn't he usually reorder blood tests during drug therapy to assess the effectiveness of the drug? This is especially true with patients who are put on blood thinner medication. If the levels within the blood are not closely monitored while patients are on these medications, they may become negatively altered and the patient can become seriously ill.

This is also the case with patients with diabetes mellitus who are taking a medication to maintain their blood sugar. These patients are instructed on how to monitor their own blood sugar levels and thereby assess the efficacy of the medication they are taking. Why should the approach to hormone therapy be any different? Laboratory testing is critical before and after initiation of any hormone therapy. Demand it of your healthcare provider! Don't be intimidated into believing you don't need occasional laboratory testing. It is essential!

What are the tests that I need?

I see so many men and women with the same complaints. Why is there so little proper laboratory investigation undertaken by physicians when it comes to patients who are on hormone therapy? Through proper interpretation of laboratory tests, most problems caused by hormone deficiency can be diagnosed and treated properly with good patient outcomes. The following discussion should help explain what tests need to be completed and how the information provided in tests can be properly interpreted by your healthcare provider.

Thyroid Tests

TSH, Thyroid Stimulating Hormone, is the hormone that comes from the human pituitary gland (see Figure One) that regulates the thyroid gland.

The pituitary gland regulates the production of the two thyroid hormones, T3 (Triodothyronine) and

T4 (Thyroxine). The scientific names are long and difficult to remember, but if you talk to a physician using the terms T3 and T4, it will be enough information for you to communicate with him. The measurement of the TSH levels in the blood is the gold standard used by physicians to identify an overactive thyroid (hyperthyroid) or underactive thyroid (hypothyroid). By measuring the TSH level, a physician can determine if the thyroid gland is making the correct amount of hormone.

If the thyroid gland is producing enough hormone, the TSH level will be within the normal range, usually a number between one and five in most laboratories. When the thyroid gland is producing too much hormone, it is said to be "overactive" or the patient is said to be hyperthyroid. If hyperthyroidism is the diagnosis, the blood level of TSH on the laboratory findings will be low (below the lowest normal number for the laboratory that does the test.)

When the thyroid gland is underactive, or not producing enough hormone, it is said to be hypothyroid. If hypothyroidism is the diagnosis, the blood level of TSH on the laboratory findings will be high, i.e., two point five or above. The higher the level of TSH, the lower the level of thyroid hormone that will be in the blood. The diagnosis of whether the thyroid gland is overactive or underactive can only be made by accurately finding the level of TSH in the blood. If the level of the two thyroid hormones, T3 and T4, is all that is checked, an incorrect diagnosis is often made and a thyroid hormone drug may be inappropriately given. In our offices, we use the guidelines of the Arestigous Endocrine Society, not the usual laboratory range of normal.

T3

Triodothyronine, T3, is one of the two hormones produced by the thyroid gland. The scientific name is a tongue-twister, so we will use short name, T3. The level in the blood of T3 is usually reported as a measurement of the total amount of this particular thyroid hormone. The correct interpretation of laboratory test results of T3 requires the physician to recognize that certain conditions (i.e., pregnancy) and certain drugs (i.e., birth control pills) will affect the test results.

The reason these conditions and drugs affect the results is that they cause the body to produce certain proteins that attach themselves to the hormone T3 and make the level appear higher or lower than the true level is in the blood. This fact makes it even more important that your physician always gets a measurement of the TSH level in your blood so that proper interpretation of the T3 laboratory value can be obtained.

T4

Thyroxine, T4, is the other hormone produced by the thyroid gland. The laboratory tests to determine the level of T4 in the blood have been available for a long time, but once again the correct interpretation of these values relies on having the TSH tested as well. To try and say that someone has too much or too little T4 in their blood can only be done by looking at the blood level of TSH at the same time. There are two tests that are used to find the amount of T4 thyroid hormone: Total T4 and Free T4. The Total T4 measures all of the T4 hormone that is currently in your blood, and the Free T4 measures the total amount of T4 hormone in your blood that is biologically available to the body. No matter which tests a physician chooses to use, the results must be interpreted only when the level of TSH in the blood is known.

Thyroglobulin Test

Thyroglobulins are the proteins that bind to and carry thyroid hormones to the tissues. Insufficient or excessive amounts of these proteins will affect thyroid hormone actions.

Thyroid Antibody Tests

Thyroid antibody tests are often for patients who develop antibodies that attack the thyroglobulin proteins or an enzyme commonly known as TPO (thyroid peroxidase) which is desperately needed for proper hormone activity. Patients who have these antibodies have a disease called Hashimoto's Thyroiditis which simply put is the body attacking its own thyroid. This is easily treated if the proper diagnosis is made. This disease is not uncommon, but often goes undiagnosed because these tests are not performed.

Below are some representative cases that provide examples of what we have just discussed:

1. T3—low, T4—normal, TSH—normal

This represents a situation commonly seen with women on birth control pills, hormone replacement Therapy (HRT), or women who are pregnant. These test results are from someone with normal thyroid function or Euthyroid. Unfortunately, it is not uncommon for this person to be treated with a thyroid hormone, which is a completely inappropriate thing for a physician to do.

2. T3—low, T4—low, TSH—high

This is a classic example of a person with low thyroid function, hypothyroidism, who needs additional thyroid hormone to regulate the thyroid function. Both thyroid hormones are low, and the TSH consequently has to be high. The pituitary is sending its messenger signals telling it to make more hormone.

3. T3—high, T4—high, TSH—low

Here is an example of a person with an overactive thyroid, hyperthyroidism. This person may need drug therapy or surgery depending on what is causing the hyperthyroidism. Both thyroid hormones are being overproduced and with these high levels the pituitary gland shuts down the production of its thyroid-regulating hormone TSH.

Far too many people are on natural thyroid supplements who don't need them. They are at risk for arrhythmia (abnormal heart rhythm) of the heart, burning out their own thyroid, and osteoporosis if the thyroid supplements are used for too long a period of time. It is imperative that patients be evaluated with the appropriate tests to determine thyroid hormone levels (T3 and T4), and have these values compared with the TSH level.

Estrogen and FSH

Estrogen is produced primarily in the ovaries. In humans, three estrogens are produced. (See Figure Three): estrone (E-one), estradiol (E-two), and estriol (E-three). The normal estrogen ratio in women is estradiol to estrone at two to one.

Please refer to Figure Three to review the following:
Estrone (E-one)—HO, H3C, O
Estradiol (E-two)—HO, H3C, OH
Estriol (E-three)—HO, H3C, OH, OH
Equilin—HO, H3C, OH

Estradiol

Estradiol is the most important estrogen in women. It is the estrogen hormone the body needs and utilizes the most and is the major hormone in a woman's system. The other estrogens are made from estradiol. If it is determined that a woman needs estrogen, she only needs her estradiol level evaluated because the body uses this to make any estrogen it needs. Therefore, request that your healthcare provider order an estradiol level for you when he orders your laboratory tests.

Follicle Stimulating Hormone (FSH)

The follicle stimulating hormone (FSH) is a regulatory hormone. A physician can learn more scientific information from the FSH level in your body than any other test. Why? The FSH level gives true meaning to what a blood or saliva measurement of estrogen indicates. Proper interpretation of the estrogen level in the body can only be achieved if the estradiol levels and FSH level are measured immediately and at the same time. The reason blood tests

Figure Three

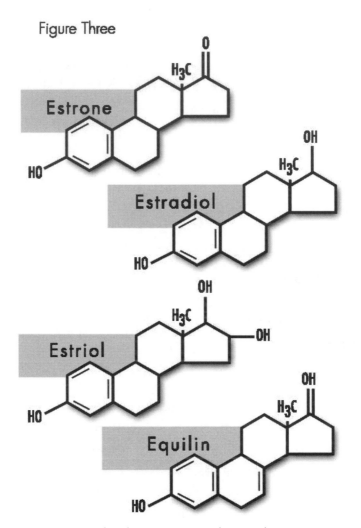

for estrogen were given a bad reputation is the results were interpreted without a proper FSH level being ascertained at the same time.

Below are some representative cases with examples of what we just discussed:

1. Estradiol—low, FSH—high (above twenty-three)

The laboratory test results of this patient show that she is estrogen-deficient and needs estrogen therapy. The low estrogen hormone level causes the pituitary gland to produce high levels of FSH which is what causes the severe menopausal symptoms women experience.

2. Estradiol—normal, FSH—high (above twenty-three)

These laboratory test results show that this patient needs estrogen, as well. This case is a good example of what many physicians and/or healthcare providers miss because they didn't order the correct blood tests or they simply don't understand the test results.

If they only had asked for an FSH level, they wouldn't have missed the diagnosis because a high FSH level indicates that the body is not getting enough estrogen.

3. Estradiol—normal, FSH—normal (less than twenty-three)

This patient needs no hormonal therapy.

CASE STUDIES

Donna, a sixty-three-year-old woman, presented to me after having undergone surgery for removal of her uterus, both tubes and ovaries at age fifty. After her surgery, she had been placed on high doses of estrogen to control her hot flashes. She told me that she never felt "right." When she told her physician that and asked to have her hormone levels checked, she was told that she was already on hormones and doing a hormone level test was useless.

I immediately ordered a hormone panel blood test for Donna as well as blood tests to measure her pituitary regulatory hormone FSH and TSH levels. The results showed that she was deficient in estrogen, testosterone, and thyroid hormone. I placed her on oral natural thyroid replacement which contained both thyroid hormone as well as estrogen and testosterone therapy with the PHDS. Six weeks later, when we rechecked her hormone levels, they had returned to the levels a woman in her thirties would possess.

Donna recently wrote to me, *"I haven't felt this good since I was pregnant twenty-five years ago."*

Note: this particular case study is an excellent example of how important proper laboratory work and correct interpretation can be in helping a physician to make the correct diagnosis. And, the therapy outcome clearly shows the power of the PHDS for delivery of precise and personal hormone treatment.

An, a forty-three-year-old woman, presented to me with a history of a complete removal of her uterus and ovaries at age thirty due to endometriosis. She was placed on the highest dose of patch estrogen which made her hot flashes "tolerable," but she often had "dryness of the vagina" which caused pain with intercourse. Since she didn't have hot flashes her physician told her she was on enough estrogen. Our blood tests demonstrated low estradiol and testosterone levels and a high FSH in spite of using hormones. Her high FSH indicated she was estrogen deficient. The lack of intercourse, due to pain, was causing problems in her marriage. Four weeks after having her pellets inserted she noticed a marked improvement in being able to sleep, think, exercise, and once again enjoy an intimate relationship with her husband. In her words: "I'm a whole woman again. I can't thank you enough."

Testosterone (Total and Free)

The testosterone level in the body is measured by obtaining both the total level of testosterone and the free level of testosterone in the blood. Why both? Because the body produces a protein—Sex Hormone Binding Globulin (SHBG)—that will render testosterone ineffective in men and women. As we discussed previously, the total level is the level that is in the blood and the free level is the amount of hormone that is biologically available to the body. The higher the SHBG activity, the lower the biologically available testosterone will be. Recent research has conclusively shown that estrogen will raise the level of SHBG in the blood and drive down the free testosterone. Both of the tests, the total level of testosterone and the free level of testosterone, are necessary to assess whether testosterone therapy is appropriate and needed.

Below are some cases with examples of what we just discussed:

1. Testosterone—normal; free testosterone—normal; FSH—normal

This patient needs no testosterone therapy.

2. Testosterone—normal; free testosterone—low; FSH—normal

Testosterone therapy is most likely indicated, but these results may mean that too much testosterone is being bound with sex hormone binding globulin (SHBG). The low level of the free testosterone indicates that there is very little testosterone available for the body to use.

3. Testosterone—low; free testosterone—low

This patient is in need of testosterone therapy.

CASE STUDIES

Patricia, a twenty-nine-year-old woman, presented to me with complaints of low energy, low sex drive and foggy thinking. She told me that these problems had existed for the previous two years since the birth of her daughter. She had seen her gynecologist regarding these complaints and the physician had told her it was all due to stress and over work and had refused to test Patricia's hormones because she was "too young to have hormone problems." She wanted to prescribe an antidepressant. When I first saw Patricia in my clinic, I ordered a hormone profile blood test and found that she had a testosterone level below twenty. I immediately placed her on testosterone PHDS therapy, and six weeks following the beginning of her treatment, she stated, *"It's a miracle; I'm not tired anymore. I have my life back."*

Edward, a forty-nine-year-old male, presented to me with complaints of no libido, poor muscle tone, and a low sex drive. His doctor at the time had measured his total testosterone and told him it was low normal and that he didn't have a testosterone problem. Our tests demonstrated his *total testosterone was low normal but his free, useable testosterone was low which validated his symptoms. Eight weeks after PHDS therapy, he had this to say:* **"It's a miracle, I can't believe the difference. My life has changed."**

I hope by reading this chapter, you have gained a better understanding of the blood tests that are necessary for a physician to make a definitive diagnosis based on scientific evidence of whether hormone replacement therapy is needed or not. Once the test results are clear he will also be better able to design a personalized hormone treatment for you, should the test show that you need it. Armed with this information, you should also be able to communicate better with your physician when speaking about hormone therapy.

Chapter 6

Traditional HRT Therapy— Side-effect Laden

*"They always say time changes things,
but you actually have to change them yourself."*
—Andy Warhol

Before we discuss traditional hormonal replacement therapy, let's review the properties we have identified as those we would like to see in the ultimate hormonal therapy. Keep these properties in mind as we review traditional HRT and you will see why they have not met your needs in the past.

The ultimate HRT should be:

- Biologically equivalent, *as close to what we have in our bodies now*
- Effective and hassle-free, *have a positive effect on reducing your symptoms and be easy to use*
- Biologically available when needed twenty-four/seven, *in your body so your glands can take what they need when they need it*

- Safe, *no liver involvement and not negative effects on other organs*
- Last up to six months, *no monthly refills or daily pill-popping*
- No increase in breast cancer, *have clear, positive clinical trial results*

An Overview of the Traditional HRT

Conjugated Estrogens

The first and most common form of estrogen utilized throughout the world (over seventy percent of the market) is conjugated estrogen (Premarin™). Conjugated estrogens are extracted from the urine of pregnant mares. If you want to use this hormone, you must accept its source. Horse estrogen is great for horses and ponies, but not for humans. The chemical structure of horse estrogen is completely alien to our physiologic system. You may be familiar with the drug names in this category—they include Premarin™, Premphase™, and Prempro™. Humans don't make a hormone called Equilin (See Figure Three), which is the prominent hormone in Premarin™. This hormone changes the normal estrogen ratio in the body, which is Estradiol to Estrone from two to one, to one to two. This reversal causes the body to be subjected to an excess of estrone, which is a very strong breast receptor stimulant.

This excess of estrone is the primary reason many women on conjugated estrogen complain of breast tenderness, water retention, and weight gain around the waist and hips. This excess could also be a factor in the increase of cases of breast cancer, after long-term usage.

To be fair, let's see if conjugated estrogen fulfills any of the properties we look for in the ultimate HRT.

- **Is it biologically equivalent?** NO! It uses Equilin, a hormone made by horses, not by humans.
- **Is it effective, hassle-free with no side effects?** NO! The use of conjugated estrogen does stop hot flashes, but often lab work demonstrates inadequate depression of FSH.

This may explain why symptoms often reappear when stress and worry arise. As for being hassle-free, you must take it every day or the effect is lost quickly.

- **Is it biologically available when needed twenty-four/seven?** NO! Oftentimes, when you need hormones at the end of the day, they may not be available (See Figure Four.) Anything taken orally produces the roller-coaster effect of rapid rise and fall. In effect, if you need hormones late in the day, you may not have sufficient levels of them for your needs—anxiety, irritability, hot flashes and insomnia may occur. This form of estrogen is not available when your body needs it.

- **Is it safe?** NO! All conjugated estrogen must be processed in the liver to be activated for the body's use. This causes a rise in clotting factors which increases the chance of clots in your veins and of pulmonary embolus (clot in the lung), which can be lethal. The safety record for conjugated estrogen in relation to breast cancer has been studied and reports have indicated an increase in occurrence if used with Medroxyprogesterone. No one should subject themselves to these risks. The other oral synthetics, Estrace™, Menest™, and Estratest™ also carry the same inherent properties as conjugated estrogen. The only difference is they have not been studied individually and may potentially be more beneficial than conjugated estrogen is.

Estradiol Patches

The next type of commonly used form of HRT estrogen is estradiol delivered in the form of a patch. Subjecting patch estrogen to the same test as conjugated estrogen yields the following results:

- **Is it biologically equivalent? NO!** It is synthetic estradiol, but derived from plant sources. Pharmaceutical companies include anything made from plants as "natural." (For example, plastics are also made from plants.) Biologically equivalent hormones are only made by small compounding pharmacies that specialize in their production.

- **Is it effective and hassle-free? NO!** Patch-delivered estradiol (PDE) is effective in controlling hot flashes, but its effect on bone reabsorption and prevention of heart disease is not well established. The only real difference in various patches is how long they last. For most patches, the primary problem is the adhesive. Many of them don't stick and if they come loose, their effectiveness ends. In addition, women often complain of the irritating nature of the adhesive on the skin, and they then discontinue the patches because of adhesive problems.

- **Is it biologically available when needed? NO!** The patch has a more prolonged effect than oral tablets but still has the roller-coaster effect. This may lead to the development of anxiety and hot flashes when at the end of its useful life.

- **Is it safe? Somewhat**. The patch allows the hormone to be absorbed; therefore, it bypasses the liver for activation. One doesn't get the increase in clotting factors, as seen in tablets. The question regarding breast cancer with regards to patches has not been specifically studied, but patches do provide a more even distribution of estradiol to estrone one to one. This is still not the natural ratio of two to one, but it is better than oral hormone replacement.

Hormone Injections

Hormone injections of estrogen and testosterone are given in the muscle and are used to treat deficiencies of these hormones. Are they the answer? NO! They are synthetic—pure and simple.

- **Is it biologically equivalent? Absolutely NOT!** No injectable biologically equivalent hormone is available. All injections are synthetic. No good things can be said of hormones given by injection into the muscle.

- **Is it biologically available when needed? NO!**
  Hormones given in injection form are absorbed in a very irregular
  fashion that causes very irregular blood levels. This is the major reason
  so few doctors use injections. Quite simply, they are unreliable.
- **Is it effective and hassle-free? NO!** Initially injections
  are effective in making symptoms go away, but long-term use is
  not possible. Increased resistances to the synthetic hormones
  build as the injections are given. Their resistance results in patients
  having to get the injections more frequently. Furthermore, these
  injections are painful and will cause scarring in the muscle with
  such frequent use.
- **Is it safe? NO!** Synthetic hormones are not safe in any form.
  Injections are the last form of therapy that should ever be used. The
  irregular absorption of these hormones causes blood levels of
  hormones to be very irregular, which in turn causes a significant
  roller-coaster effect. Never allow your physician to use injections!

Equivalent Hormones

As we know, biologically equivalent hormones are the closest to our own natural
hormones and definitely a better way to go than the synthetic drugs. Recently more
physicians are having biologically equivalent hormones made in special pharmacies, which are called compounding pharmacies. Pharmacies can hand make
custom compound hormones for patients who ask for them. This has been the best
development in hormone therapy in a long time. However, it is not only the type
of hormone that is prescribed that matters, but the delivery system for that hormone
that matters just a much. The problem with other forms of delivering hormones are
they need to be swallowed, applied as a cream, or administered in sublingual
(under the tongue) tablets. These will give you peaks and valleys of your
hormone levels in the blood, meaning it causes you to have ups and
downs with your hormones and your symptoms.

Balance is key when it comes to hormone replacement therapy. This
estrogen ratio in addition to a proper level of equivalent testosterone is
what returns a woman's body to normal physiology.

Men, on the other hand, who produce only miniscule levels of estrogen in their bodies, need only testosterone supplementation to achieve balance and return to their former selves—optimum well-being.

Using the same test questions that we used for traditional HRT, let's look at how equivalent hormones rate.

- **Is it biologically equivalent? YES, thankfully.**
- **Is it effective and hassle-free? Not really if applied to the skin or taken as pills.** The hormones that are compounded from individual components and administered through capsules, creams, or sublingual tablets don't necessarily relieve the majority of patients' symptoms at low doses. Usually they have to be taken twice a day to be effective and they can be expensive, as well. In addition, the doses taken have to be high to be effective—five to ten milligrams a day, which equates to one hundred to three hundred milligrams each month. This is a lot of hormone, but it is necessary for some women to "feel better." The use of these forms of hormones is labor intensive for patients, especially if they are using creams. The creams are messy and expensive and have a very short useful life in the body. This often leads to frequent use or under use which results in the return of all the problems. The sublingual tablets are placed under the tongue and may take a long time to dissolve if not made properly. They often need to be taken twice daily for proper hormone levels. The problem with sublingual is the compounding pharmacies must be experienced in their production or a useless tablet is produced.
- **Is it biologically available when needed? NO!** These forms of therapy all produce the same roller-coaster effect that all short-acting tablets, patches and cream-delivered hormones generate.
- **Is it safe? YES!** Biologically equivalent hormone is the one form of hormone that is safe. The safety is increased if it is absorbed

E2 Level Pills, Patches vs. Pellets

Figure Four

Smith R/ Studd, J WW
Brit Jour Hosp Med, 1993, Vol 49, No 11

directly into the bloodstream. In other words, don't swallow it; absorb it (cream or sublingual tablets). No increase in breast cancer has been shown thus far with the use of biologically equivalent hormones.

The Pellet Hormone Delivery System for Delivering Equivalent Pellet Hormones

PHDS therapy, using equivalent hormone pellets, consists of placing tiny estradiol and testosterone pellets painlessly under the skin in the fatty tissue. These pellets are similar to the size of a grain of rice for women. The effects of each implantation can last from four to six months or even longer. The hormone levels achieved through PHDS therapy are the closest thing to natural hormone levels produced by the human ovary and testes (See Figure Four.) The hormone levels achieved are constant, steady, and predictable. No other form of hormone delivery can produce a consistent blood level of estradiol and testosterone.

Hormone pills, whether natural or synthetic, produce a "roller-coaster" effect (See Figure Four.) The pills give high levels of hormones two to four hours after ingesting them and the levels decrease steadily after that. In some individuals, their hormone levels may be so low twelve hours later that they need to take another dose, but are not permitted to do so by prescription limitations. Once-a-day pills are absolutely the farthest thing from the natural rhythm of hormonal secretion. The ovary and testes are designed to secrete hormones twenty-four hours a day. PHDS therapy in the form of hormone pellets is the only type of hormone replacement therapy that recreates the body's natural hormone-producing rhythm. The use of pills and patches can never recreate the hormone levels achieved through PHDS therapy. More importantly, pills or patches cannot respond with increased dosages of hormones when the body requires more. In contrast, by using PHDS therapy hormone is always available for the body to take whenever it is needed, no matter what amount is required. This property alone distinguishes the PHDS therapy from other types of HRT and puts it in a category far superior to that of pill or patch usage in recreating a balanced hormonal environment. Release of hormones from pellets is consistent and controlled by heart rate—the faster or slower the heart beats, the faster or slower the hormone is released.

Clearly, from what you have just read, you can see that estrogen or testosterone hormonal deficiencies are well corrected by PHDS therapy by using estradiol and testosterone pellets.

I have summarized a few of the proven benefits of PHDS therapy:

1. PHDS therapy uses equivalent hormones; therefore, normal levels of each hormone are achieved in the blood utilizing the lowest possible dosage of each hormone.

2. PHDS therapy releases hormones directly into the blood stream, bypassing the liver and avoiding serious side effects with other organs.

3. PHDS therapy is the only form of hormone therapy that can release hormone on-demand, twenty-four hours a day, seven days a week, when the body requires it.

4. PHDS therapy is made of pure crystallized, biologically equivalent estradiol and testosterone.

Pellets are equivalent in structure. They are nothing like the synthesized hormones manufactured by pharmaceutical companies. The equivalent hormone pellets used in the PHDS are both natural and biologically equivalent to the estrogen and testosterone your own body once produced in correct amounts.

The pellets are derived from soy and other natural plant-based ingredients. They are hand-formulated in compounding pharmacies and possess the exact hormone structure of the human hormone estradiol (estrogen) and testosterone. Female pellets themselves are smaller than the size of a grain of rice.

Using the test questions, let's look at how they rate.

- Is it biologically equivalent? YES!!!
- Is it effective and hassle-free? YES!!
- Is it biologically available when needed? YES!!
- Is it safe? YES!!! Biologically equivalent pellet hormones are one form of hormone that is safe. The safety is increased as they are absorbed directly into the bloodstream. No increase in breast cancer has been shown thus far with the use of biologically equivalent pellet hormones.

Progesterone

Progesterone is one of the hormones in our bodies that stimulates and regulates various functions. It plays a role in maintaining pregnancy. The hormone is produced in the ovaries, the placenta (when a woman gets pregnant) and the adrenal glands. It helps prepare your body for conception and pregnancy and regulates the monthly menstrual cycle.

During the reproductive years, the pituitary gland in the brain generates hormones— follicle-stimulating hormone (FSH) and luteinizing hormone (LH) that cause a new egg to mature and be released from its ovarian follicle each month. As the follicle develops, it produces the sex hormones, estrogen and progesterone, which thicken the lining of the uterus. Progesterone levels rise in the second half of the menstrual cycle, and following the release of the egg (ovulation), the ovarian tissue that replaces the follicle (the corpus luteum) continues to produce estrogen and progesterone.

Estrogen is the hormone that stimulates growth of the uterine lining (endometrium), causing it to thicken during the pre-ovulatory phase of the cycle.

One of progesterone's most important functions is to cause the endometrium to secrete special proteins during the second half of the menstrual cycle, preparing it to receive and nourish an implanted fertilized egg. If implantation does not occur, estrogen and progesterone levels drop, the endometrium breaks down and menstruation occurs.

If a pregnancy occurs, progesterone is produced in the placenta and levels remain elevated throughout the pregnancy. The combination of high estrogen and progesterone levels suppress further ovulation during pregnancy. Progesterone also encourages the growth of milk-producing glands in the breast during pregnancy.

High progesterone levels are believed to be partly responsible for symptoms of premenstrual syndrome (PMS), such as breast tenderness, feeling bloated and mood swings. When you skip a period, it could be because of failure to ovulate and subsequent low progesterone levels.

The word "progestogen" or "progestin" refers to any hormone product that affects the uterus in much the same way as our natural progesterone. Effective synthetic versions of progesterone, called progestins, have been around since the 1950s. A micronized capsule version of natural progesterone (from soy) was developed more recently.

Progestogens are included along with estrogen in combination oral contraceptives and in menopausal hormone therapy. Progestins are also used alone for birth control, and for treatment of a variety of other conditions including abnormal uterine bleeding and amenorrhea (absence of periods); endometriosis; breast, kidney or uterine cancer; and loss of appetite and weight related to AIDS and cancer. Progestins may also be used as a diagnostic aid to check the effects of estrogen.

Progesterone is an important hormone, but it's been given almost mythical status. |According to John Lee, M.D., in his book, *What Your Doctor May Not Tell You About Menopause*, published in May 1996, it can resolve the majority of perimenopausal and menopausal problems women face. He and others tout natural progesterone as a bone builder and a perfect alternative to estrogen. This is only partially correct. The use of progesterone cream has expanded dramatically in the United States since he published this book. Outside of the United States, where pellet hormones are commonly used, the application of natural progesterone cream is infrequent or is completely ignored. Why the disparity in the use of progesterone between the United States and other countries? Why do physicians in other countries prefer to use natural estradiol and testosterone rather than natural progesterone?

Clinical research does not support progesterone as the "wonder hormone." For women and men, progesterone production occurs as a transitional stage on the way to making estradiol and testosterone. (See Figure Two.) This simple diagram shows exactly what the body does with progesterone. Progesterone does not perpetually reside in the body nor does it have all the effects the public is led to believe. In fact, progesterone is only produced in substantial amounts in a non-pregnant woman's body for ten days of each month, and daily production of progesterone is seen only during pregnancy. Women who breast-feed do not produce progesterone.

The clinical research reports quoted in many books are based on research done with synthetic progesterone, progestin, which is not natural progesterone. Frankly, the research done using natural progesterone has been very disappointing. One example is a study performed at St. Luke's Hospital in Bethlehem, Pennsylvania by Helene B. Leonetti, MD and others, Transdermal Progesterone Cream for Vasomotor Symptoms and

Postmenopausal Bone Loss. The study results presented at the 2004 Twelfth Annual World Congress on Anti-Aging in Las Vegas, Nevada, decisively demonstrated that topical progesterone cream at ten times the strength of the creams recommended by John Lee, M.D., and others, (which is twice the prescription strength normally ordered), produced no bone growth after a year of usage by a large study group of women.[4] Based on this information, progesterone cream does not appear to be the wonder treatment it has been advertised to be. Research also shows that the same cream is not nearly as effective as it is reported to be as a protector against heart disease, stroke, Alzheimer's disease, and osteoporosis.

The History of Pellets

In 1935 women in Europe were given hormone therapy by the insertion under the skin of estrogen and testosterone in the form of pellets. This form of therapy was developed as a means to supply hormones to young women who had undergone a complete hysterectomy and became a very successful form of delivering estrogen and testosterone therapy. The therapy was then provided for women who had not undergone a hysterectomy and also showed excellent results as long as progesterone was given at the same time. Based upon all the data and discussion in the previous chapters, man-made, bio-equivalent hormones that either have to be swallowed, injected, or topically applied, are not consistently effective, are burdened with many negative side effects, and do not provide consistent, evenly distributed hormones.

The best form of biologically equivalent hormone replacement is one that is directly absorbed into the bloodstream and delivers hormones on demand when your body needs them just as the ovaries and testes do. With more than a decade of research and over twenty-six years of experience, the pellet hormone delivery system (PHDS) has been proven to be far superior to other forms of biologically equivalent HRT on the market. The usage of pellets for hormone replacement has been in the United States since 1939.

Let's make sure that we clearly understand the difference between bio-equivalent and equivalent. Equivalent means biologically equivalent to what your body produces both in structure and action. The definition of natural (compared to the synthetic materials used by the pharmaceutical companies) is a hormone made from a plant source. In order for a hormone to be truly equivalent, it needs to have the precise, biologically-equivalent chemical structure of the human hormone, not simply a laboratory-created chemical equivalent. Human bodies need and want equivalent hormones to replace what they have lost or are unable to produce. Hormones lost by aging or surgery must be replaced or augmented with equivalent hormones to ensure that the problems such as night sweats, sleep disorders, decreased sex drive, anxiety, irritability, and many others, do, in fact, lessen or cease completely. In 1935, hormone pellet insertion for menopausal women in Europe was created. In 1939 Robert Greenblatt, M.D. introduced this therapy to North America.

Why Don't All doctors Use the PHDS?

At this point you may be asking yourself, if this therapy is so superior, why isn't it widely utilized in the United States? The primary reason is lack of exposure through marketing and advertising. A further reason pellets have not been widely utilized is the simple economic fact that the formula cannot be patented. This means that pharmaceutical companies cannot monopolize a market and, therefore, cannot generate significant profits. Consequently, the machinery of marketing and physician-training has been kept relatively small. "Implants bypass the liver, avoiding the first-pass effect on liver metabolism of the hormone. This prevents the unphysiological ratio of oestradiol [estradiol] to oesterone [esterone] found with oral preparations."[16]

"Oral estrogen results in minor increase in clotting studies consistent with recent studies showing no improvement in heart attack and stroke, because of their 'First Pass' through the liver."[17]

"Oral preparations, unlike implants, also reduce liver metabolism of clotting factors and lipids."[18]

Further Reasons to Use PHDS Therapy

Let's look at PHDS therapy in relation to the use of synthetic hormones and also the way hormones are administered. We have already established that estradiol and testosterone levels in the human body need to exist in sufficient quantities to satisfy the body's needs. The question is, how much hormone needs to be given to achieve normal (physiologic) levels of each hormone? If one tries to achieve normal human levels with pills, a significant amount of hormone must be given. For example, the smallest dose of oral estrogen hormone available is zero point three milligrams of Premarin. This means that if you took Premarin, you would take in a minimum of nine point seventy-five milligrams of estrogen hormone monthly (thirty days times zero point three milligrams). If you took Estrace at zero point five milligrams daily, you would receive fifteen milligrams monthly. Compare this to the estradiol delivered through PHDS therapy, at zero point five milligrams to three milligrams monthly. Only estradiol patches at a dosage of zero point zero two five milligrams, can deliver such low amounts of estrogen as do pellets in the PHDS therapy, but not steadily. They still give highs and lows of hormone levels.

You are probably wondering why pills have to be given in such high doses. The reason is that hormones given orally have to be processed in the liver to be activated. This process is termed "first pass metabolism," which is the passage of a substance through the liver cells in order to activate or deactivate the substance. This requires activation of an enzyme system in the body of the cell. The substances are released into the bloodstream along with their byproducts. This then causes stimulation of other substances in the liver to be produced such as clotting factors. These substances can have a damaging effect on the liver cells themselves causing scarring and possibly a loss of liver function.

The oral hormone has to be given in such high doses to compensate for the predictable loss of hormone in the liver and the loss of usable hormone in the intestinal tract from lack of absorption. Consequently, high doses need to be given so that only a fraction of the hormone taken in by the body ever finds its way into the bloodstream and is available for supplying hormone to satisfy the body needs. The balance of the unused hormone remains in the liver or is lost in the stool. The high doses of estrogen also produce the unwanted effects of breast tenderness, over-stimulation of the estrogen receptors of the breast tissue, and significant weight gain and fat deposits. It also destroys the natural distribution ratios of estrogen in the blood. This can add to the unwanted side effects produced by oral hormones.

A question you may be asking is, why swallow a hormone when the body prefers to absorb it? The manufacturers of oral synthetic hormones have no real answers. Pellets are produced by pharmacies and pharmaceutical companies in Europe and many other nations. Why is production of pellets suppressed in the United States? Apparently, it is not as profitable as producing oral medications, and the public is not as aware of pellets as it is of oral drugs. Why would a person use anything else if they were as well-informed about pellets as they apparently are about oral synthetic hormones? As you can now see, the method of absorption profoundly influences the effect of estradiol and testosterone in the human body. Why then shouldn't these hormones be given in a way that is nearly equivalent to the way the body releases hormones into the bloodstream?

Remember that the hormone FSH regulates the flow of estrogen in the body. The human body desires the steadiest and most consistent hormonal level possible even when confronted with physical or emotional stress. The human body regulates the levels of allsecreted hormones to deal with these changes, both external and internal, that affect the secretion of hormones in the human body. The only form of hormone delivery that can recreate what the body does naturally is a hormone delivery system such as PHDS therapy.

The type of hormone pellet used in the PHDS therapy, be it estradiol or testosterone, is a tiny, solid cylinder (approximately three millimeters in diameter), about the size of a small grain of rice. The skin is first prepared by numbing it with a small amount of Novocaine, similar to the numbing effect you receive from the dentist. The pellets, which are cylindrical in shape, are placed under the skin with the use of a needle instrument that is inserted into the fatty tissue. The outer surface of this cylinder is the active area of hormone delivery. A small percentage of each pellet's surface area is released on a daily basis over a twenty-four hour period. This steady secretion keeps the level of hormones consistent in the bloodstream. The entire procedure takes less than a few minutes. Best of all, the procedure is completely pain free.

But what happens if you exert significant physical demands upon your body, such as exercise? Or what occurs when you experience emotional stress, such as a surprise visit from your supervisor or in-laws? If you are taking oral hormones or are wearing a patch, you will most probably be left without the appropriate hormonal reserves because pills, patches and shots cannot provide your body with the hormones needed immediately. Estradiol and testosterone pellets, like the type used in PHDS therapy, can do this because the increase in heart rate and muscle activity will generate a faster release of hormone from the surface area of the pellet, thereby releasing more hormones. When the stress ends, the body returns to its normal heart rates and activity and the release of hormones returns to its usual level. PHDS therapy is the only option which enables your body to access hormones when it needs them. More importantly, this can be reproduced many times throughout the day and no oral tablets, shots or creams can do this.

The hormone patches cannot respond quickly or provide sufficient hormone to satisfy what the body needs immediately. What the human body needs to correct a hormone deficiency is the biologically equivalent hormone it lacks. This is common sense. Doesn't it seem right that the human body would prefer using an equivalent hormone to the one it provides naturally? Of course it would. Synthetic hormones (bio-equivalent), whether made from plants or animal products, are just reasonable facsimiles. "Testosterone pellet implants have many of the ideal features of a long-acting androgen depot [storage], including being safe, highly effective with stable clinical and biochemical effects, economical, providing flexible dosing, and excellent long-acting properties due to a near-zero-order dissolution. A single biodegradable implant of six hundred to twelve hundred milligrams provides stable, effective, and well-tolerated replacement for four to six months and pellets can provide excellent androgen replacement in most physiological settings."[19]

In summary, if a person is deficient in estradiol or testosterone, replacing that hormone with the equivalent hormone it needs, delivered in the equivalent secretion pattern, such as through PHDS therapy, would be the logical choice. To further bolster this statement, the scientific research that supports the use of pellets as a replacement delivery system for estradiol and testosterone has been continuously published and documented since 1939. In fact, the use of pellets like the type used in PHDS therapy has been employed in the United States since 1939 and they can only be made in a compounding pharmacy.

It's amazing to me how much this treatment modality has been ignored by the physician training programs in the medical schools in the United States. Of course, research money is, in great part, supplied by pharmaceutical companies. What company wants stiff competition against the products it produces and promotes? It seems that a solution this simple would be available to everyone, but the opposite is true. There are very few practitioners using this form of therapy. Why? Physicians are never exposed to this in specialty training because they are schooled only in the "traditional" forms of hormone therapy.

Chapter 7

Precise and Personal—Nature's Answer for You

"One cannot dance well unless one is completely in time with the music,
not leaning back to the last step or pressing forward to the next one,
but poised directly on the present step as it comes."
—From *Gift from the Sea*, Anne Morrow Lindbergh

The balanced state within your body is not the same as my balanced state or anyone else's for that matter. Achieving that individual balance is no easy matter, and a physician must take the time to scientifically uncover the secrets for each one of us and then apply the proper therapy to achieve the personal balance. The trend today among women and men, more than ever, is for "natural" forms of hormone replacement therapy. This desire has stimulated patients to seek out physicians who not only use natural hormones, but specifically, equivalent hormones. These physicians take special care to design personalized therapy for each of their patients. Hormone levels are different for each one of us and the therapy must also be personalized.

PHDS therapy is based on a thorough understanding of how the human endocrine system works and what it needs to maintain balance.

Once your hormone levels are accurately measured and analyzed, you will receive the proper dose of PHDS hormone pellets to fulfill your own body's requirements. Your hormone levels will thereafter be periodically checked in order to assess the ongoing success of your hormone replacement therapy. There is no guesswork or "one size fits all" with PHDS therapy. PHDS is designed specifically for each individual patient.

Just like the natural hormone delivery system your body is accustomed to, the PHDS estrogen and testosterone pellets, once implanted, work automatically. The hormones are secreted in tiny amounts into the bloodstream daily. When more hormone is needed due to stress or exercise—the body will respond and deliver more. The release of the hormone is controlled by a patient's heart rate. A higher heart rate delivers more hormone.

When you are under stress or perform exercise, you require higher levels of estrogen and testosterone to function optimally. Simply put—your body has a built-in response system that calls for just the right amount to be released. When your ovaries (in women) and testicles (in men) were functioning properly, it was their job to produce hormones and release them in correct amounts into the bloodstream.

In menopause and andropause, the ovaries and testicles slow down their production of estrogen and testosterone until they reach a point where they are unable to keep up with the demands of the body.

The PHDS pellet therapy is able to pick up where the ovaries and testicles left off and let the pellets work in partnership with your body to provide for its needs. Any rise in your heart rate will cause increased blood flow over the pellets, releasing the needed amount of hormone into your bloodstream. In the case of exercise, an increased amount of estrogen released from the muscles being exercised will also cause a release of hormone replacement pellets.

Scrutiny of clinical data reveals that numbers of women do not respond to traditional "hormone replacement therapy" dosing. The usual clinical response is to increase the dose of prescribed estrogen without re-evaluating the reason for the ineffectiveness of the hormone therapy. Every woman responds uniquely to a given dose (and possibly route) of estrogen therapy, and response will vary with the organ systems involved. Technology now provides a distinction between "healthy women" who are experiencing a natural reproductive transition and "patients" who have latent or overt disease. This biologic, evidence-based approach allows physicians to decide on the need for hormone therapy, the dose that should be prescribed, and the patient's response to her treatment over time.[20]

What Is Individualized Therapy?

Medicines that work wonders for some can be totally ineffective for others— sometimes even toxic.

Equivalent hormone replacement therapy is used to help treat the symptoms of menopause, perimenopause, and postmenopause. Treatment with equivalent hormones usually includes creating a unique cocktail of hormones for the individual patient, based on hormone deficiencies identified via focused blood testing. These are often referred to as "custom-compounded" hormone products. The major benefit of this type of treatment is that doses are individualized, and the mixture of products may not be commercially available.

Within the next chapter, I will address some of the very serious health issues that plague individuals who, for one reason or another, have become hormonally deficient. You will see that hormonal therapy is a precise and personal goal for each patient and physician. Restoring the body back to its natural hormonal balance will help instill a greater sense of well-being and normalized body functions. Through this we address the serious health issues that we often see with our patients.

Chapter 8

Alleviating Serious Health Issues

"And if things don't looks so cheerful just show a little fight.
For every bit of darkness there's a little bit of light."
—The Bluebird of Happiness

Menstrual Migraine

Migraine headaches can affect anyone of any age but are particularly troublesome for women in the reproductive years, when occurrence patterns are tied to the menstrual cycle. The International Headache Society defines menstrual migraine as a migraine headache that affects a woman each month between the second day before the start of the menstrual period and the end of menstruation. Menstrual migraine is different from non-menstrual attacks of migraine, even in the same women, in the regularity of its timing and its greater severity. Compared with other times in the menstrual cycle, a migraine is more than twice as likely to occur during the first three days of menstruation and more than three times as likely to be severe.

Migraine headaches are more common in women, and sixty percent to seventy percent of women with migraines report some relationship with their menstrual period. Usually there is an increased frequency before, during and after menses. There is a category of migraine that is called a true menstrual migraine. This is a migraine headache that occurs regularly each month but only between the second day before the menses and the end of menstruation. Menstrual migraine is thought to occur in about fourteen percent of women.

Levels of female sex hormones, specifically progesterone and estrogen, sharply decline in the late phase of the menstrual cycle, just before the onset of the period. Studies have shown that supplemental estrogen given at the time of the natural monthly decline in these hormones delays the onset of migraine until the estrogen level finally decreases. These findings suggest that estrogen withdrawal may trigger migraine in women who are predisposed to migraine.

In a 1970 issue of the *Journal of Neurology*, BW Somerville, MD, reported on a study that found women who developed headaches prior to and during their menstrual periods

responded favorably to estrogen therapy.[21] I wanted to explore the viability and impact that estradiol pellets might make on menstrual migraines, so I began treating women of all ages who were suffering with menstrual migraines with PHDS therapy. In all cases, a small dose of pellet estradiol was inserted under the skin, and within three to seven days estrogen levels were elevated, but more importantly, the estradiol levels were higher during the premenstrual and menstrual period and the occurrence of patients' headaches was reduced significantly or eliminated completely. I have treated women from age twenty-two to age forty-nine who are suffering with menstrual migraines by using PHDS therapy, and the results were over ninety percent success in eliminating their headaches. For anyone who is incapacitated with this form of migraine headache, PHDS of estradiol can be a savior for you. Further evidence of this was found in Dr. Magos's study which eliminated headaches in twenty out of twenty-four patients.[21]

CASE STUDIES

Meredith, an eighteen-year-old woman, presented to me with a history of suffering from incapacitating migraine headaches that began with the start of her monthly period and lasted for seven days. She was bedridden during these episodes and required narcotic pain relievers to help with relief from the headaches.

She related a history of these headaches since age thirteen when she began to have regular menstrual periods. When I first saw Meredith, I immediately ordered hormone panel blood tests before her periods and again during the headaches. The results showed a substantial drop in her estrogen levels during the headache periods.

I began therapy with the PHDS of low dose estrogen and the severity of her headache was immediately reduced during her next period that occurred two weeks after start of therapy.

Joanne, a thirty-eight-year-old mother of two, presented to me with a history of only suffering true migraine headaches at the time of ovulation (when estrogen rose to high levels) and when she had her menstrual period (when her estrogen was very low). I began treatment with enough estrogen through the PHDS to stop the highs and lows of estrogen and establish a balance of estrogen in her body. Her headaches ceased immediately and she remains headache-free to this day. As Joanne said, **"I can take care of my family without using drugs to stop my pain."**

Ovarian Cancer

Ovarian cancer is the most commonly fatal of gynecological cancers, affecting one in forty-eight women. It is a type of female cancer that is, unfortunately, most commonly diagnosed in its advanced stages. Early-stage tumors are usually not found, which is when they are most treatable and curable. Current treatment involves surgery and chemotherapy, but most ovarian cancers return within two years.

There is scientific evidence that birth control pills can be used as a preventative treatment for ovarian cancer. The most compelling argument is found in the research that demonstrates that birth control pills effectively reduce the incidence of ovarian cancer: "The protection afforded by oral contraceptives against ovarian cancer appears to be independent of the dose of estrogen or progestin," as reported by Dr. Roberta Ness of the University of Pittsburgh and colleagues in 2000. In the study, approximately eight hundred women with ovarian cancer were compared with more than thirteen hundred women who did not have cancer. Overall, women who used birth control pills had a forty percent lower risk of developing ovarian cancer. The risk was further reduced the longer the duration of oral contraceptive use.[26]

In June of 2007, *Science Daily* reported the results of a study showing that hormone therapy can extend life in ovarian cancer patients. The study, originally published in the journal, *Clinical Cancer Research*, proved that the targeted use of an anti-estrogen hormone could prolong the life of some patients by up to three years and delay the use of chemotherapy in others. John F. Smyth, Professor of Medical Oncology at the University of Edinburgh, who led the research program, said: "This is an important landmark in the research and treatment of ovarian cancer. Despite intense scientific research over the past twenty years, there have been few new leads in our understanding of how this disease operates. But this study suggests that the addition of hormone therapy to our treatment strategy could extend and improve the lives of women with cancer."

Dr. Simon Langdon, senior lecturer in cancer research at the University of Edinburgh and the lead scientist behind this trial, said: "Ovarian cancer can be a devastating disease, so this new discovery is particularly exciting."

This sounds wonderful, but how is it possible? The answer, I believe, lies in the extremely low levels of FSH (follicle stimulating hormone) that birth control pills produce which keep the ovaries quiet and inactive. With this information taken into account, the primary goal for physicians should be to keep the FSH level in *postmenopausal* women as low as the levels produced by birth control pills. The hormones in birth control pills are synthetic, and the biologically-equivalent estradiol that suppresses the

FSH continually and as effectively as birth control pills is found in estradiol pellets. Oral forms and creams do not suppress the FSH. (Elevated levels of FSH continually bombard the ovary with stimulation. Therefore, it stands to reason that decreasing stimulation by FSH reduces the chance of developing ovarian cancer). During the ten-year period from 1992 to 2002, there have been no documented cases of ovarian cancer among the nine hundred and seventy-six patients in the study group I have treated with PHDS therapy. All of these patients have very low FSH levels. In summary, if we don't allow the ovary to be stimulated, we can reduce the chance of ovarian cancer. The only form of equivalent hormone that accomplishes this is estradiol PHDS therapy.

Post Partum Depression

It is not out of the ordinary for women to experience mood changes during pregnancy. The moodiness is generally caused by fluctuations in hormone levels. Many of these mood changes are normal and even expected, since having a baby can lead to several lifestyle changes. Support from family and friends is helpful at this time.

Approximately fifty percent to seventy percent of women may experience depression for a short time after pregnancy. These are usually feelings of anxiety, irritation, tearfulness, and restlessness that are often called "the post-partum blues." This generally occurs in the first few weeks after pregnancy and goes away soon without the need for treatment. However, post-partum depression is a more serious condition that affects between eight percent and twenty percent of women after pregnancy, especially during or at four weeks. It is essential that medical attention be sought immediately for women to treat post-partum depression. Women who are more prone to post-partum depression may have or have had one or more of the pre existing conditions:

- Mood or anxiety disorder prior to pregnancy, including depression with a previous pregnancy
- A close family member who has had depression or anxiety

- Something stressful happened during the pregnancy, including illness, death or illness of a loved one, a difficult or emergency delivery, premature delivery, or illness or abnormality in the baby
- Are under age twenty
- The pregnancy was not planned or is not wanted
- Currently abuse alcohol, take illegal substances, or smoke (these are also serious medical health risks for the baby)
- Have little support from family, friends, and a significant other
- Have a poor relationship with your husband, boyfriend, or significant other or are unmarried
- Previously attempted suicide
- Have financial problems (low income, poor housing)
- Received poor support from your parents in childhood

How is PPD recognized?

Most of the symptoms are the same as in major depression. In addition to depressed mood, the following symptoms may be apparent daily:

- Negative feelings toward the baby
- Lack of pleasure in all or most activities
- Decreased appetite
- Loss of energy experienced
- Feeling withdrawn, socially isolated, or unconnected
- Feelings of worthlessness or guilt
- Agitation and irritability
- Trouble sleeping
- Difficulty concentrating or thinking
- Thoughts of death or suicide (a suicide plan)

There is no single test to diagnose post-partum depression. If the above symptoms are obvious, a discussion with a physician should take place immediately to review potential treatment. Sometimes depression following pregnancy can be related to other medical conditions. Hypothyroidism, for example, causes symptoms such as fatigue, irritability, and depression. Women with post-partum depression should have a blood test to screen for low thyroid hormones.

Post partum depression (PPD) is a devastating disease that can develop shortly after the wondrous miracle called birth. It frequently goes untreated and can have disastrous results for mother, baby, and the entire family. How does post partum depression develop and can it be prevented? The obvious answer is that the body, just after the placenta is removed, is robbed of all of its hormone (estradiol, progesterone and testosterone) production. Therefore, the goal would be to effectively elevate the hormone levels with equivalent estradiol.

PPD causes significant distress to a large number of women; the demand for effective therapies to treat PPD is considerable. Estradiol therapy has a prophylactic effect in women at high risk for developing PPD. The prevention of a decline in estradiol levels may prevent the onset of PPD. Studies also suggest that estradiol has antidepressant effects in women and may provide a safe and effective alternative to traditional antidepressants in women with PPD. Clinical trials are ongoing to further substantiate the use of estradiol to prevent PPD.

The use of equivalent hormones delivered through PHDS therapy poses no threat to infants who are breastfeeding. If it did, then breastfed babies of mothers who have started menstruating again would have problems because menstruating breast feeding mothers are producing all their hormones. The only form of therapy that can do this safely is PHDS therapy because of the extremely low levels of hormones utilized. Furthermore, this hormone is absorbed directly into the bloodstream and the liver is bypassed, making it safe for mother and child. The best part is that it begins to work in thirty-six to seventy-two hours after it is administered. Think of the number of women whose post-partum suffering could be eliminated. This therapy does not interfere with antidepressant medications.

CASE STUDY

Kirsten, a twenty-seven-year-old mother of two, had delivered a baby by C-Section four months prior to coming to see me. She developed severe depression within two to three weeks of her delivery and could not care for her baby without help. Her husband and mother, concerned about her, took her to a psychiatrist for therapy and she received an antidepressant which caused her to become sleepy and lethargic. She came to me for a second opinion, and I found her estradiol level as well as her testosterone level was very low. I treated her with estradiol pellets and testosterone pellets and she also remained on her antidepressant medication. At her post recheck appointment, six weeks later, she stated: **"I could see a difference in four to five days. I have more energy and feel more normal. I am also on half the antidepressant I was on before."**

Osteoporosis

The *Merck Manual of Health and Aging* reports that "in the United States, about eight million women and two million men over age fifty have osteoporosis. In millions of other women and men over fifty, bone density (mass) is low but not low enough to be considered osteoporosis. These people have osteopenia (which means deficient bone). They are at risk of developing osteoporosis as they grow older."

The oldest therapy for the elimination of osteoporosis is estrogen replacement therapy. There are as many deaths from complications of osteoporosis as there are from breast cancer. Osteoporosis needs to be treated aggressively, and synthetic hormone therapy must be avoided.

According to the National Institutes of Health (NIH), "If you think you're at risk for osteoporosis or if you're menopausal or postmenopausal, you may want to ask your doctor or other health care provider about having a DEXA II-scan (dual-energy X-ray absorptiometry). It measures spine, hip, or total body bone mineral density, or how solid bones are. The results can show the presence and severity of osteoporosis, or if you're at risk of developing it or having fractures. You can prevent osteoporosis. The key steps are to follow an eating plan rich in calcium and vitamin D and be sure to get regular weight-bearing exercise. Although food sources are usually better absorbed, calcium and vitamin D intake can be taken as supplements, but check with your healthcare provider first. Too much of either can cause problems. Recommended daily intakes of calcium and vitamin D are given in Box Fourteen. Good food sources of calcium include canned fish with bones (such as salmon and sardines), broccoli, dark green leafy vegetables, (such as kale, turnip greens, and collards), dairy foods such as nonfat or low-fat milk, calcium-fortified orange juice, soy-based beverages with added calcium, and cereal with added calcium. Vitamin D is made by the body—being in the sun twenty minutes a day helps most women make enough. But it's also found in foods such as fatty fish (sardines, mackerel, and salmon), and cereal and milk fortified with Vitamin D.

Thirty minutes of weight-bearing exercises such as walking, jogging, stair climbing, weight training, tennis, and dancing, done three to four times a week, can help prevent osteoporosis. It's also important not to smoke and to limit how many alcoholic beverages you drink. Too much alcohol (for women, more than one alcoholic drink a day) can put you at risk for developing osteoporosis. Smoking increases bone loss by decreasing estrogen production. Osteoporosis is treated by stopping bone loss with lifestyle changes and medication. Hormone therapy has been used to prevent and treat osteoporosis.

J.W. Studd demonstrated that oral estrogen increases bone density only one to two percent and patch estrogen increases bone density three point five percent, but estradiol pellets elevate bone density eight point three percent annually.[22] "*...oral oestregen [estrogen] in general increases vertebral bone density by approximately one to two percent per annum(29) whereas the seventy-five milligram oestradiol [estradiol] implant, which achieves oestradiol [estradiol] levels in general at least double those of oral therapy, has been shown to increase vertebral bone density by eight point three percent per annum.*"[25] If a therapy is to be used, it should be safe and easily tolerated. No safer estrogen is available than equivalent estradiol, delivered through PHDS therapy. Therapy is the best way to deliver it to the bone. Estradiol PHDS therapy is absorbed directly into the bloodstream and none is lost. No other form of providing estrogen to the body can deliver such doses at continual, steady levels, which is necessary for optimum bone growth. This is why estradiol pellets have been an important mode of therapy for osteoporosis in the United Kingdom since 1990. In fact my wife, who developed osteoporosis at forty-three years of age, was found to have normal bone density after six months of PHDS therapy without any other medications.

Vaginal Atrophy and Dryness

A very frequent complaint from women is vaginal dryness which causes pain with intercourse. The atrophy (thinning) of the vaginal lining and loss of muscle tone from the lack of estrogen and testosterone in post-menopausal women may produce profound physical and emotional problems for them and their significant others. The thinning of the vagina causes dryness, loss of lubrication, and pain with intercourse from the trauma produced by excess friction. The loss of muscle tone accelerates the development of uterine prolapse and urinary incontinence.

Uterine Prolapse

If you have uterine prolapse, it means that your uterus has tilted or slipped. Sometimes it slips so far down that it reaches into the vagina. This happens when the ligaments that hold the uterus to the wall of the pelvis become too weak to hold the uterus in its place. Uterine prolapse can cause feelings of pressure and discomfort and urine leakage may be noticed as well.

How Is Uterine Prolapse Treated?

Treatment choices depend on how weak the ligaments have become, your age, health, and whether you want to become pregnant. Surgery is sometimes recommended.

Non surgical treatment recommendations may include:
- Exercises (called Kegel exercises) can help to strengthen the muscles of the pelvis. Kegel exercises: Tighten your pelvic

muscles as if you are trying to hold back urine. Hold the muscles tight for a few seconds and then release them. Repeat this exercise up to ten times for up to four time each day.

- Taking estrogen to limit further weakening of the muscles and tissues that support the uterus.
- Wearing a pessary—a rubber, diaphragm-like device— around the cervix to help prop up the uterus.

As uterine prolapse progresses loss of support increases for the bladder, and rectum, it frequently leads to necessary surgery to correct the problem that accompanies its development (urinary and rectal incontinence, excess pelvic pressure). The use of estradiol PHDS therapy and testosterone therapy treats both of the problems safely. The estradiol thickens the vagina, and the combination of estradiol and testosterone allows the muscles to thicken and tone. The use of PHDS therapy together with proper exercise can help one to avoid surgery.

Chronic Fatigue Syndrome and Fibromyalgia

According to the Centers for Disease Control and Prevention (CDC), chronic fatigue syndrome (CFS), once thought by some doctors to be a psychological problem or even an excuse for malingerers, is a real disease that affects more than a million Americans. Early diagnosis and treatment of the disease are important for recovery. "CFS (chronic fatigue syndrome) is a terrible illness that prevents many people from taking part in everyday activities and participating in the things they enjoy," CDC Director Dr. Julie Gerberding said. Up to eighty percent of people with chronic fatigue do not know they have it, the CDC said. Its causes are unknown but it can cause profound exhaustion, sleep difficulties, and problems concentrating and remembering.

Flu-like symptoms, including pain in the joints and muscles, tender lymph nodes, sore throat and headaches are also common. "A distinctive characteristic of the illness is a worsening of symptoms following physical or mental exertion," the CDC said. "Diagnosis is primarily made by taking a patient's medical history, completing a physical exam and lab tests to rule out other conditions," it added.

"The CDC considers chronic fatigue syndrome to be a significant public health concern, and we are committed to research that will lead to earlier diagnosis and better treatment of the illness," Gerberding said. Scientists do not know the exact prevalence of CFS because the disorder is so hard to define. The CDC estimates that up to half a million people in the US have the symptoms of CFS, but have not been diagnosed by a doctor. The chronic fatigue and immune dysfunction syndrome (CFIDS) Association of America (www.cfids.org), a patient support group, estimates the number to be about eight hundred thousand. They estimate that ninety percent of people with CFS have not been diagnosed and are not receiving care.

Because CFS is so hard to define, some physicians still believe that it is not a real disease, but is psychological in origin. However, the National Institute of Allergy and Infectious Diseases recognizes CFS as a serious illness, and the Centers for Disease Control and Prevention (CDC) have developed criteria to define it.

The following are some possible causes of CFS:

- *Viruses and other germs.* Many patients develop CFS after an illness resembling a viral infection, and researchers first believed that a virus was the cause. Epstein-Barr virus, which causes mononucleosis, was especially suspect. However, scientists have been unable to link CFS with any specific agent as the single cause. They are trying to discover whether any infectious organisms play a partial role in causing CFS.
- *Immune system disorders.* Some research has found that people with CFS have either overactive or underactive immune systems. However, these people do not have the diseases that are usually associated with overactive immune systems, such as lupus and rheumatoid arthritis, and they are not more likely to develop cancer or infections, as may people with depressed immune systems.
- *Brain abnormalities.* Studies show that people with CFS have abnormally low brain levels of a hormone called corticotropin,

which helps in coping with stress. These people often report that they were under a great deal of stress just before the condition began. Scientists think that, due to the low hormone levels, their immune systems might overreact to stress, causing the symptoms of CFS. However, CFS patients who were given a replacement hormone that restored their hormone levels to normal did not get better. This result suggests that low hormone levels do not directly cause CFS.

- *Blood pressure disorders.* Some evidence suggests that CFS is related to a blood pressure disorder called neutrally mediated hypotension (NMH), in which the brain signals the heart to slow down when you stand up. Your blood pressure falls, temporarily depriving your brain of oxygen, so that you become light-headed and may even faint. Many people with CFS have such symptoms when they stand for long periods, and scientists are testing whether the medicines given to people with NMH might also help those with CFS.

CFS can begin in different ways. Aside from fatigue, people with CFS experience a variety of other symptoms such as difficulty concentrating, sore throat, and muscle aches that either persist or come and go for more than six months. CFS often begins after you have had a cold, an intestinal virus, or bronchitis. Teenagers and young adults sometimes get it after a bout of mononucleosis. Other people find that CFS starts during a period of high stress. But for some people it comes on slowly, and there is no distinct, triggering event. You feel too tired to carry out your normal daily routine, and may be easily exhausted by any activity.

Early in the illness, the most common symptoms are sore throat, fever, muscle pain, and muscle weakness. At this point you may sleep a great deal, but as time passes you may instead have difficulty falling asleep, or may wake up too soon.

Scientists do not know the exact prevalence of CFS because the disorder is so hard to define. The CDC estimates that up to half a million people in the US have the symptoms of CFS, but have not been diagnosed by a doctor. The chronic fatigue and immune dysfunction syndrome (CFIDS) Association of America (www.cfids.org), a patient support group, estimates the number to be about eight hundred thousand. They estimate that ninety percent of people with CFS have not been diagnosed and are not receiving care.

No one therapy works, but reducing stress, dietary restrictions, gentle stretching and nutritional supplementation have all been shown to help. Drugs are sometimes prescribed.

Chronic fatigue syndrome (CFS) and fibromyalgia are two diseases that affect many people. I often find elevated levels of antibodies to the Epstein-Barr virus which causes mononucleosis in adolescents and chronic fatigue in adults. I also often find low testosterone levels in both chronic fatigue and fibromyalgia patients and have used PHDS therapy with testosterone pellets to correct the hormone deficiencies, resulting in increased energy and a better quality of life. The traditional antidepressant therapies used for both need to be continued, but adding testosterone helps these patients regain a better quality of life.

CASE STUDY

Julie, a thirty-nine-year-old female, was diagnosed with chronic fatigue syndrome (CFS) at the age of thirty-five. She was always tired and had to give up exercising because of her fatigue. The stress was too much for her anymore. She took the children to school and then came home to rest. Her husband had to do the majority of the housework and her best friend, who I had previously treated for CFS, brought her to see me. She had been told by her physician that there really was nothing else to be done and she would have to learn to deal with it the best she could.

Her blood work demonstrated that she was in menopause, a fact her physician ignored due to her youthful age, and she also had a low testosterone level. I began therapy with estradiol pellets, testosterone pellets, and biologically equivalent progesterone to protect her uterus. A few weeks after pellet therapy began, she reported back, "I now feel more energized and have returned to my routine of working out. My husband likes the new woman in the house!"

Patients with HIV or AIDS

Low testosterone levels are common in both men and women with human immunodeficiency virus (HIV) infection and may contribute to loss of lean body mass and AIDS wasting. Many patients who are affected by HIV or AIDS often complain of fatigue and lethargy.

Many HIV-positive men are treated with synthetic testosterone to give them increased energy. Why utilize synthetic testosterone when biologically equivalent testosterone is available? With so many drugs utilized in the treatment of HIV and AIDS, the liver needs to be protected. Synthetic testosterone does not afford this protection, but testosterone pellets do give this protection. My male patients feel stronger and have a better quality of life and better physical strength.

In addition to its effects on body composition, testosterone treatment results in improved mood and libido in HIV-infected women and increased bone mineral density in HIV-infected men.[30]

Breast Cancer

Previously in this book, we discussed the results of the WHI Study concluding that the development of breast cancer with the use of oral conjugated estrogens and synthetic progesterone was found to increase breast cancer after ten years.(1) But in fact, biologically equivalent hormones could be breast protective. The best form of biologically equivalent hormone that gives normal levels of estradiol to the breast tissue is estradiol HPDS. In a study I have completed with nine hundred and sixty-seven women who took part in the study from 1992 till 2002 using PHDS therapy, there has been only one case of breast cancer. Forty percent of this group of women was taking biologically equivalent progesterone as well. Theoretically, in this ten-year period, there should have been over one hundred cases of breast cancer, because the incidence of breast cancer in women of all ages is one out of nine. Therefore, if one out of nine women will get breast cancer whether they are taking hormones or not, you would think that over one hundred of my patients would have developed breast cancer. My explanation as to why this happened is that estradiol pellets release a tiny amount of hormone daily, a biologically equivalent hormone, and does not produce excess stimulation of the estrogen receptors in the breast. From looking at the above numbers, you could easily say that the form of estrogen replacement therapy might be breast protective. Another consideration is the patient who has had breast cancer. What can be done to improve her quality of life? Too often these patients suffer with severe hot flashes, loss of libido, mood swings and generally not feeling like they once did. The use of testosterone PHDS therapy for improving their problems has been very successful. D.Gambrill, MD, who has been using estrogen and testosterone pellets to treat breast cancer patients, has recently published a paper focusing on the safety of PHDS therapy. The results of his study were excellent and the data shows less cancer reoccurrence in patients using PHDS therapy than patients not using pellet hormones.[23] Research continues to identify the effectiveness of hormonal therapy in breast cancer management.[24]

Insulin Resistance

The National Diabetes Information Clearinghouse (NDIC) defines insulin resistance, "Insulin resistance, a generalized metabolic disorder, is a silent condition that increases the chances of developing diabetes and heart disease." Insulin resistance is the basis of the hormonal cause of overweight women and men. And, the reverse of this is—hormone therapy, diet and exercise are the answers to menopausal and andropausal fat accumulation problem.

I often hear my patients complain that, "I've put on all this fat around my middle." This sort of statement is as common in men as in women when they are experiencing menopause or andropause. They also tell me, "I diet, exercise, and do all the right things, but I'm still gaining weight and putting on fat!"

While this is usually the case and they are doing everything they can to maintain health and weight through proper diet and exercise, it is often not enough and thus causes extreme frustration.

Why does this happen to us as we age? As the body enters a time during the normal aging process when it can no longer sustain adequate levels of estrogen and testosterone for women and testosterone for men, the impact throughout the endocrine system is profound.

Without the proper levels of these hormones, especially testosterone, the entire metabolic system breaks down. Before we begin an in depth discussion of insulin resistance, let's review the metabolic system and its importance within the body.

The Metabolic System

The metabolic system manages the chemical and physical changes that take place within the body. These changes allow our bodies to grow properly and function normally at all times. Metabolism, not just something as simple as gaining or losing weight, is a process that involves the breakdown of complex organic components of the body in order to produce energy needed for all of the bodily processes to work at full capacity. It also allows the building up of complex substances, which forms the material of the tissues and organs. Actually, metabolism is a collection of chemical reactions that takes place in the cells of the body to convert the fuel in the food we eat into the energy needed to power everything we do, from moving to thinking to growing. Specific proteins in the body control the chemical reactions of metabolism, and each chemical reaction is coordinated with other body functions. Metabolism is not just one process, but thousands of metabolic reactions that all happen at the same time and are regulated by the body to keep all of the cells healthy and working.

Metabolism is a constant process that begins when we're conceived and ends when we die. It is a vital process for all life forms—not just humans. If metabolism stops, a living thing dies.

When the metabolic system is sick or not functioning properly, it is called metabolic syndrome (or the insulin resistance disorder), defined by the American Heart Association as being characterized by a group of metabolic risk factors in one person. They include:

- Abdominal obesity (excessive fat tissue in and around the abdomen)

- Atherogenic dyslipidemia (blood fat disorders—high triglycerides, low HDL cholesterol and high LDL cholesterol—that foster plaque buildups in artery walls)
- Elevated blood pressure
- Insulin resistance or glucose intolerance (the body can't properly use insulin or blood sugar)
- Prothrombotic state (e.g., high fibrinogen or plasminogen activator inhibitor–one in the blood)
- Proinflammatory state (e.g., elevated C-reactive protein in the blood)

The dominant underlying risk factors for this syndrome appear to be abdominal obesity and insulin resistance. Insulin resistance is a generalized metabolic disorder, in which the body can't use insulin efficiently. This is why the metabolic syndrome is also called the insulin resistance syndrome.

Other conditions associated with the syndrome include physical inactivity, aging, hormonal imbalance and genetic predisposition.

How Is the Metabolic Syndrome Diagnosed?

The American Heart Association and the National Heart, Lung, and Blood Institute recommend that the metabolic syndrome be identified as the presence of three or more of these components:

- Elevated waist circumference:
  Men—Equal to or greater than forty inches (one hundred two cm)
  Women—Equal to or greater than thirty-five inches (eighty-eight cm)
- Elevated triglycerides:
  Equal to or greater than one hundred fifty mg/dL
- Reduced HDL ("good") cholesterol:
  Men—Less than forty mg/dL
  Women—Less than fifty mg/dL

- Elevated blood pressure:
  Equal to or greater than one hundred thirty/eighty-five mm Hg
- Elevated fasting glucose

If testosterone is absent, the muscles decrease their uptake of glucose and the body struggles to maintain its normal levels of glucose and insulin. The result is the development of "insulin resistance."

Insulin resistance, IR, is becoming rampant in our society, but goes underrated. Young women, even in their teens develop a disease called Polycystic Ovarian Syndrome which results in marked weight gain, acne, abnormal hair growth, irregular periods and infertility because of insulin resistance. Older women more commonly deposit increasing amounts of fat through the waist and hips. Men develop the classic "beer gut" and/or "love handles."

How Does the Process of Insulin Resistance Start and What Can Be Done to Stop It?

Our bodies, as they age, become less functional as we lose our capability of maintaining the hormone levels we enjoyed in our twenties and early thirties. As testosterone levels decline the muscles have a tougher time of taking glucose from the blood and burning it. As glucose levels rise from lack of being able to burn sugar, the body will produce increasing amounts of insulin. This increase in insulin will trigger the transformation of glucose into fat and triglycerides. The presence of normal testosterone levels in both men and women helps prevent their insulin resistance. Testosterone stimulates the muscles to uptake and burn glucose rapidly, thereby reducing sugar levels in the blood causing insulin secretion to remain normal. When testosterone is absent, the muscles are inefficient utilizers of glucose, insulin rises and fat begins to be deposited. This can happen rapidly or develop slowly and steadily over a period of time. That's when I hear patients complain: "I diet, exercise, and I still get fatter!" Without testosterone, exercise produces cardiovascular protection but no fat burn. If you can't burn fat, you deposit it, and insulin resistance causes the deposition of fat not only under the skin but also in the abdominal cavity.

The fat in the abdominal cavity called "*visceral fat*" is the worst. Visceral fat substantially raises the possibility of high blood pressure, cholesterol and triglyceride elevations and diabetes. This process will continue until the cycle is broken. Breaking the cycle of insulin resistance takes a multifaceted approach. The diagnosis should be suspected when fat develops around the middle, blood pressure begins to rise, and cholesterol and triglycerides start to rise. Careful monitoring of all these factors is needed with blood pressure checks, measuring the "true" waistline, and getting your cholesterol and triglycerides checked regularly.

Concerning blood pressure, when the readings start rising by ten points over your usual reading, and even if you are still below the one hundred thirty/eighty range: start paying attention! When you start feeling your pants and skirts getting tight around the waist, start measuring. If the waistline in a woman exceeds thirty-two to thirty-three inches and forty inches in a man, you probably have I.R. The level of severity may vary from mild to severe, producing metabolic syndrome to Type II diabetes. Another clue is the gradual rise of cholesterol and triglycerides in the blood even if your levels are "in the normal range" when they begin to rise and your diet and exercises haven't changed, it may be the I.R. starting to rise.

Insulin resistance (IR) is the underlying cause of Metabolic Syndrome, Type II Diabetes, and Polycystic Ovarian Syndrome. After you realize what it does you can just look at someone and know they have it. They have large amounts of fat around their waist and hips and a beer gut. I would venture to say you will see at least forty to fifty percent of the population in the United States walking around with the external appearance of someone with IR

If you have it, what do you do for it? You simply must change everything starting from the "inside out"; testosterone levels must be returned to "real" normal levels. Testosterone creams, gels and shots do no produce the steady continuous levels of testosterone the body needs to reverse insulin resistance. They instead cause spikes of testosterone that actually worsen insulin resistance. Only the pellet hormone delivery system (PHDS) can reproduce the steady levels of testosterone in the blood that are so necessary for proper uptake of glucose by the muscles and increasing insulin sensitivity (IS). In addition you need more testosterone during exercise and stress or the glucose released from the liver during exercise will not be utilized by the muscle as well and the glucose will be used, but no fat will be burned. This is what leads to continued fat deposition in spite of regular exercise. Only PHDS therapy allows the body to increase its testosterone level "on command" and decrease it during periods of low muscle activity. If someone is using shots, creams, or gels, they cannot in any way adequately regulate or create the steady levels of testosterone necessary to make the body more insulin sensitive during exercise and keep it insulin sensitive during periods of low muscle activity such as sitting, meditating, or sleeping. Wouldn't it be comforting to know that your body is doing its job without having to think about it! The PHDS therapy works continuously to keep the body balanced and normal.

Exercise to be productive and burn fat must be done with intensity. If walking down the street talking with your exercise buddy is viewed as enough to burn the excess fat in your body, you're very mistaken. If you're not breathing heavily and unable to talk easily, your exercise intensity is insufficient to "burn fat." Short periods of intense exercise done twice a day, or more often, will allow you to burn more fat than you would if you were just "walking" for exercise. You can walk for thirty to forty minutes at your regular pace and if you're not "huffing and puffing" you are not burning fat. You are getting cardiovascular benefit, but little fat burn. You would burn more fat by walking very rapidly for ten minutes at a pace that makes you swing your arms rapidly to produce huffing and puffing, twice or three times daily in the morning, at lunch time or before dinner. Remember if huffing and puffing, you are burning fat and getting even more cardiovascular benefit. If you don't want to lose your exercise buddy who just wants to "vent" during your walks, convince them to substitute four or five two- to three-minute periods of intense walking during the period and talk in between. The intensity of the exercise is more important than the duration. Additionally, if you complete this period of exercise just before a meal, you will also burn those incoming calories. This doesn't mean you get a candy bar as a reward!

Diet is an important tool in reducing insulin resistance. But if your hormone levels are not balanced, dieting is more likely to fail or the weight just comes rushing back. If you're not normal internally and if you are taking in the wrong foods, you worsen your insulin resistance. As an example one large slice of pizza will make you insulin resistant for four to six hours—four to six hours of increasing fat deposits. Regular alcohol intake in excess of one glass of wine or beer a week will worsen insulin resistance. If you have IR now, until you have reversed it by balancing your hormones with the PHDS, exercising, and decreasing the amount of alcohol and simple carbohydrates (anything made with white flour or sugar) you take in, you'll never become normal and healthy.

Anyone who has IR must be very careful with their intake of carbohydrates or the pancreases will over secrete insulin. If this happens and you are resistant to its effects, it will turn your blood glucose into fat and it will become deposited inside your abdomen and around your waist. A diet low in carbohydrates, especially simple carbohydrates, is the key. Take in twenty percent to twenty-five percent of your diet in complex carbohydrates such as whole grains. If you like the taste of pizza, top your salad with cheese and pepperoni or get a small slice on a whole wheat crust. You will only be insulin resistant for one and a half to two hours with a whole wheat crust. But bear in mind if you don't have a steady release of testosterone your muscles will not be induced to uptake the glucose normally and burn it to produce muscle health and energy. To put it simply, you cannot maximize the benefits of diet and exercise and reverse insulin resistance without having normal testosterone levels continuously. The only alternative is to take certain medications given to diabetics to increase their insulin sensitivity. In my practice we also give these medications, but couple this with testosterone pellet therapy to maximize the effects of the medications.

An ideal program for anyone who is insulin resistant might be to have truly normal testosterone levels—a diet consisting of fifty-five percent protein, twenty-five percent carbohydrates and twenty percent fat coupled with proper amounts of good quality, intense exercise.

CASE STUDY

Tom, a forty-five-year-old police officer, presented to me complaining of increasing fatigue coupled with a rise in his weight, an increasing waistline which went from thirty-five inches to forty-one inches, and rising blood pressure. He was tested and found to have a slight elevation in his fasting glucose, cholesterol, and triglycerides. His primary doctor had found this earlier and told him to diet and exercise. He told me he was getting too tired to exercise, and when he did he was unable to recover for two to three days.

I found not only the high glucose and fats, but also a very low total and free testosterone along with an underactive thyroid. He was treated for his testosterone deficiency with testosterone pellets and given natural thyroid (Nature-Throid®). In ten to twelve weeks he had regained his energy, was able to exercise and noted a ten-pound weight loss. But more importantly, he had a two-inch loss in his waist. The words he used were: **"I'm back! I can't believe it!! I am back to me!!"**

The restoration of steady testosterone levels to what a man would have in his thirties as well as correcting his hypothyroidism restored his insulin sensitivity and normal metabolism. Thyroid hormone and testosterone aid each other in maintaining a normal metabolic environment.

CASE STUDY

Anita, a fifty-five-year-old female, presented to me with complaints of hot flashes, fatigue, poor exercise tolerance, slow recovery from exercise and no libido, which was worsened by dryness of the vagina. Her gynecologist did not do hormone levels, but instead told her: "I know what your problem is, you don't need blood work. Just take these hormone pills and if one pill doesn't take care of your hot flashes and vaginal dryness, take two pills a day." She did as she was asked and noted her weight increased rapidly when she went to two pills daily. She went down to one, but her hot flashes returned.

When I evaluated Anita, we did blood tests and found her to have a low estradiol in spite of taking pills; a high FSH which accounted for her hot flashes and moodiness; and zero testosterone which caused her lack of libido, weight gain and fat. She had a thirty-eight inch waistline, fat hips, slightly elevated blood pressure. Her cholesterol was two hundred twenty-nine, and her triglycerides were one hundred sixty.

*Her diagnosis was very evident: estradiol and testosterone deficiency with insulin resistance. With her high cholesterol and triglycerides, I immediately started her on our program of estradiol and testosterone pellets delivered through the PHDS and encouraged two periods of walking briskly for ten minutes each morning and evening. She was also instructed on how to maintain a low carbohydrate eating plan. Six weeks after her initial treatment she returned and her words were: "**My hot flashes were gone in three to four days, and I can sleep again. I've lost one and a half inches in my waist, but my weight hasn't changed. My husband said to give you a hug for the new sexy woman I am.**"*

Anita is a classic case. She had insulin resistance, hormonal imbalance, and metabolic syndrome. Her repeat laboratory results at six weeks were: total cholesterol one hundred eighty-five; HDL from four hundred sixty to forty; triglycerides one hundred ten, blood pressure of one hundred twenty-eight/seventy-eight from one hundred thirty-eight/eighty-six and she had regained her well-being and sex life. The reason this all took place is that her testosterone once again was able to activate her muscles to accept glucose more readily, thereby decreasing her insulin resistance. She lost inches around her waist and hips, but little weight loss occurred because the testosterone caused her muscles to grow and burn fat.

Remember: Muscle Weighs Thirty-three and a Third Percent More Than Fat!!

To conclude, we have discussed in this chapter one of the most widespread disease processes in the United States today. It is grossly underdiagnosed and often poorly treated. Just giving medicine to decrease insulin resistance and not treating the hormone deficiencies that are present only does half the job.

You should suspect insulin resistance if you're a woman with a waistline between thirty-two and thirty-four, (eighty percent of women with a waistline thirty-four inches or over have insulin resistance; or eighty percent of men with a waistline of forty inches have insulin resistance). Elevated blood pressure comes with it or greater than seventy-seven percent chance of having insulin resistance. High cholesterol and triglycerides or slight elevation of a fasting blood sugar also substantially increase the presence of insulin resistance. Most importantly a combination of any two of these three factors indicates a one hundred percent diagnosis of insulin resistance.

Chapter 9

The New You—
A Look Into
the Crystal Ball

"The empires of the future are the empires of the mind."
—Sir Winston Churchill

When we began this book, we created a list of how you should optimally feel with a properly balanced hormonal system. In light of all that has now been said, we should create a new list, a list of how great you should feel with a properly balanced hormonal system.

After having taken so many pills for so long, it may seem almost impossible that just a few rice-sized pellets, like the type used in PHDS therapy can actually provide all that your body needs. Because they are not ingested into your stomach, then processed by your liver, many of the flavorings, buffers, and excess "medicines" are not required. When your body is low in either estrogen or testosterone, it seeks a source, finds what it needs from the pellets, processes it and utilizes it immediately. Because of this, people using PHDS therapy:

- Feel like they have regained control of their bodies and their lives
- Sleep more consistently and soundly without sleep problems
- Have a renewed interest in sex
- Realize greater mental clarity
- Enjoy renewed vitality and zest
- Are more enthusiastic
- Are calm, relaxed and stable
- Achieve better results with exercise (less effort more results)
- Secure additional benefits like increasing their bone mass (as much as four times greater than oral hormones)
- Experience reduced menstrual migraines
- Reduce their fears about breast cancer because PHDS therapy does not stimulate breast tissue, as compared to synthetic hormones.

The only form of therapy that satisfies the body's hormonal needs is subcutaneous (under the skin) estradiol and testosterone PHDS therapy.

Let's summarize what we have learned about PHDS therapy:
- Are they biologically equivalent? Yes! The hormones are derived from soy, and more importantly, hand-compounded to be the biologically equivalent human form of estradiol and testosterone. The body has what it can no longer produce.
- Is it effective and hassle-free? Yes! The PHDS therapy is the only form of hormone therapy that effectively reduces levels of FSH to normal. The elevation of FSH in women and men causes anxiety, irritability, hot flashes, lethargy and loss of well-being. The other forms of therapy require high doses of hormones to affect this. Pellet hormone therapy requires minute amounts of hormones to effect the lowering of FSH.
- Are they biologically available? Yes! The pellets, once implanted, work automatically.

The hormones are secreted in tiny amounts daily and when more hormone is needed during increased stress or exercise, the body will receive more hormone. This is caused by the rise of the heart rate causing increased blood flow over the pellets and in the case of exercise increased thermal release from muscles being exercised. No other form of hormone administration can do this. PHDS therapy is hassle-free and can last from four to six months. The quality of life that is given back to patients utilizing PHDS therapy is second to none. I know this because I hear it many times a day and use testosterone PHDS therapy myself.

- Is it safe? Yes! PHDS therapy hormones are biologically equivalent and absorbed directly. Therefore, no liver involvement is necessary. The hormones also don't interfere with medications for heart disease, high blood pressure, kidney disease, or thyroid disease. Biologically equivalent hormone does not increase the risk of breast cancer. The only difference between PHDS therapy for men compared to women is the amount of hormones needed. Men consume more testosterone; women consume estrogen and testosterone. The amount of time between treatments is the same, the procedure is the same, and most importantly, the overall positive results are the same. With PHDS therapy, men will realize:

- A restored sexual drive
- Relief from hormone-related depression
- Consistency—no more roller-coaster effect compared to oral therapies, injections, creams or gels
- Elevated energy levels
- Greater capacity for getting in shape
- Increased mental clarity and focus
- Decreased body fat
- Improved erectile ability
- Improved mental clarity, focus and concentration

Do Diet and Nutrition Really Matter in Achieving Hormonal Balance and Optimal Health?

The answer is yes, and I'd like to spend some time providing you with a thorough understanding of how diet and nutrition absolutely do matter in attaining a goal of optimal health.

First of all, you need to know and understand a couple of facts pertaining to nutrition and its impact on hormone balance:

1. If an imbalance in thyroid hormones, adrenal hormones, testosterone, the estrogens (estrone, estradiol, estriol), and/or progesterone exists within your body, your immune system will be affected.
2. Our own chemical environment (within our bodies) and our own nutrition are both contributing factors to hormone imbalance.

According to Dr. Robert Atkins and others, "Poor nutrition can cause ill health and suppress immune function."

- Nutrients will not be present in your body if you don't provide the proper food or nutritional supplementation that the body needs to function.
- If your digestive system is threatened at all, it will not be able to complete its task of breaking down food into the proper form for the body to use. And thus, the supports that the body needs to function (the immune system) will not be available.

In his book, *Nature's Answer to Drugs*, Dr. Robert Atkins stated, "Virtually every study comparing supplement takers with a matched group that does not take supplements shows that those taking nutrients are far healthier."

Vitamins and minerals, also called micronutrients, are obtained by eating vegetation and animals that make them. Minerals come from the earth and if the soil that plants are grown in is lacking in minerals, so will the plants be lacking in minerals. Our bodies do not make minerals, we must provide them. Micronutrients "function principally as coenzymes (in collaboration with enzymes) for a variety of metabolic reactions and biochemical mechanisms within our many bodily systems. Each enzyme is specific to one biochemical reaction. Enzymes are catalysts that speed up specific chemical reactions that would proceed very slowly without them," as discussed by Elson Haas, MD in his **Staying Healthy** book series. Without micronutrients, our bodies would suffer deficiency diseases, an abrupt decline in health and eventual death. According to

Dr. Earl Mindell, "Micronutrients regulate our metabolism through enzyme systems. A single deficiency would endanger the whole body."

Carbohydrates, protein and fats, also called macronutrients, are where we get our energy. The micronutrients in our bodies help to convert the macronutrients into forms our bodies can use. Without macronutrients, our bodies would suffer malnutrition, starvation, and eventual death.

The following is a list of nutrients that support immune function: [31]

- Zinc—supports the thymus gland, which trains the T-cells in the immune system
- Iodine—supports activity of natural killer cells
- Vitamin C—increases antibody production
- Vitamin E with vitamin C—increases T-cells, interleukin 2, and TNF
- Vitamin A—normalizes cell division and supports the thymus gland and antibody production
- Selenium—supports T-cell activity, NK cells and antibody production
- CoQ-Ten—supports one-gG antibody production
- Glutathione—supports T-cell activity
- B6—supports T-cells and B-cells, plus fifty other enzyme reactions
- Antioxidants (plant nutrients)

In 1997, the following appeared in the Journal of the American Medical Association: "The era of nutrient supplements to promote health and reduce illness is here to stay…There is overwhelming evidence of immunological enhancement following such an intervention."[32]

While we're very aware how easy it is today to add supportive vitamins, minerals and antioxidants to our diet to make sure we cover any deficiencies, we must be careful not to confuse deficiencies and providing optimal micronutrient additions.

Having the proper balance of vitamins and minerals in our bodies is very important, as we discussed above, but we have to be careful not to have too much of any one vitamin because research has shown that an excess of one vitamin might cause the same symptoms as the deficiencies would.

It is more important to ensure that the proper vitamin supplementation is designed to create stronger vitamin function by combining specific vitamins than simply taking more of one or the other.

We've talked about nutrition supplements, such as vitamins and minerals and how they can definitely enhance the immune system. Now let's talk specifically about what nutritional elements each of the glands within the endocrine system needs to function properly.

The Thyroid

Iodine is an element found in food such as seafood, and added to supplements and salt; it is essential to the body for the manufacture of thyroid hormone. Should you take iodine supplements if you have a thyroid problem to ensure that your body has enough iodine?

The thinking behind taking iodine or kelp supplements is that in many parts of the world, goiters and thyroid disease are related to iodine deficiency. In the United States and other developed countries, iodine deficiency is not very common anymore, due to the addition of iodine to salt—iodized salt—and other food products. In fact, the most common forms of thyroid disease found in the United States are autoimmune thyroid diseases like Graves' Disease or Hashimoto's Thyroiditis, and these have nothing to do with iodine deficiency.

Actually, thyroids are extremely sensitive to iodine, and you need to be careful about *adding* too much iodine to the diet as it can irritate or aggravate the thyroid. Most doctors say not to worry about some iodized salt, or the iodine present in a food item such as an occasional sushi dinner. Stephen Langer, author of *Solved: The Riddle of Illness*, the follow-up book to Broda Barnes' *Hypothyroidism: The Unsuspected Illness*, advises **against** taking iodine or kelp supplements for people with autoimmune thyroid disease.

Women need to focus on nutrition. We know that nutrition is involved in approximately half of the ten leading causes of death in women—coronary heart disease, cancer, stroke, diabetes, and diseases of the liver and kidneys. The incidence of osteoporosis and extremes in body weight are approaching epidemic proportions in women. Nutritional education is a must for all women. "As female 'baby boomers' enter midlife in record numbers, more and more of them are becoming aware of the link between what they eat and their health and longevity," reports Joan Pleuss, RD, MS, CDE, CD, bionutrition research manager at the Medical College of Wisconsin. She also states, "...a number of issues emerge that require changes in the nutrients we need."

The federal government's general Dietary Guidelines for Americans describe a healthful diet this way: "Start with plenty of breads, cereals, rice, pasta, vegetables, and fruits. Add two to three servings from the milk group and two to three servings from the meat group. Remember to go easy on fats, oils and sweets, the foods in the small tip of the Pyramid."

Here are some important nutritional considerations for menopausal and post- menopausal women as recommended by national nutritional specialists [51]:

- Cardiovascular disease and omega-three fatty acids—fish and shellfish are rich in n-three fatty acids and are known to have beneficial effects in cardiovascular disease. They also have a tendency to lower blood pressure. Two to three fish meals per week along with a low-fat diet are beneficial.
- An elevated level of a compound called homocysteine in the blood has been linked to cardiovascular disease. Elevated

levels are associated with poor intake of the B-vitamins, including folic acid, vitamin B-six and vitamin B-twelve. Look for foods that are rich in these B-vitamins whenever possible.

- One study has shown that postmenopausal women who consume at least one serving of whole-grain products daily reduce their risk of heart disease by about one third in comparison to those who rarely eat any whole grain products.
- Bone health and osteoporosis—nutrients or food components linked to bone health include calcium, vitamin D, magnesium, copper, iron, zinc, boron, vitamin C, and vitamin E. Vitamin D is responsible for helping the body absorb calcium. Magnesium also helps the body absorb both vitamin D and calcium, while copper, iron and zinc are important for bone development and structure. Zinc and vitamin E are antioxidants, while copper helps to keep bones from thinning. Boron works with magnesium and vitamin D to enhance calcium absorption.
- Alcohol, caffeine, warm beverages, and spicy foods can bring on hot flashes. Carefully monitoring what triggers a hot flash and moderating intake is advisable.

In summary, diet is extremely important for men and women alike as is regular exercise. So, avoid excess calories, exercise every day (an hour of physical activity is recommended), eat fewer trans fatty acids, limit fat consumption, and maybe add some soy-rich foods, which studies show can help to diminish menopause symptoms.

Here are just a few of the hundreds of testimonials I have received from patients who have regained their hormonal vigor through PHDS therapy:

"I tried it all, Premarin™, patches, creams, you name it! No matter what I used, I stillfelt just as bad. After PHDS therapy, my life began!"
—Mrs. Patty from California

"Thank you for changing my life. At age thirty-eight I am feeling like eighteen again and a lot happier."

—Mrs. Elmira from California

"I had a hysterectomy six years ago. My friend said I had been scaring her with my mood swings and instability. Now I'm me again! My husband even says he can see the young woman he married twenty years ago."

—Mrs. Deborah from California

"For the first time since my hysterectomy in 1989, I actually feel so wonderful. I felt bad for so long I forgot what it was like to have lots of energy, no leg cramps, no night sweats, be able to think straight, be able to sleep all night, and to have sexual desires again. I am a new woman!"

—Mrs. Patty from California

"After working thirteen hours on Monday and fourteen hours on Tuesday from being a floor nurse, I got home last night and I wanted sex out of the blue. My husband was expecting a cranky worn out nurse and got a thirty-five-ish wow-mamma. I feel thirty-five."

—Mrs. Judi from Kansas

"For five years I have tried every combination of hormone replacement therapy to treat my symptoms, to no avail. With each passing year my symptoms of night sweats, huge temperature shifts, sleeplessness and depression were getting worse. I found that menopause was definitely not for sissies! I was anxious to try anything. With the PHDS Therapy, I couldn't have hoped for a better outcome. Within two weeks I was sleeping through the night with NO night sweats. My temperature comfort zone has normalized. I can't describe what a difference it has made in my quality of life. I would recommend PHDS therapy to anyone who is ready to live life normally again!"

—Ms. Carol DDS, MS from California

"I just wanted to let you know how much better I felt almost immediately after I had my first PHDS Therapy treatment. I actually felt peppier, I have slept better, been much more patient, and had much more energy. I also used to have headaches almost every day, many times all day long. But now I find I hardly ever take any pain medication for them. My hormone levels were much improved after three weeks. I look forward to feeling this good for a long time."

—Mrs. Eileen from California

"For five years, I took testosterone shots and used adhesive patches. Because I am an active person, the patches did not stick, and besides, they just didn't give me enough help to make them worth the hassle. The shots made my hemoglobin shoot way up. That is not what I wanted. What I really wanted was something that was a lot more permanent, less bothersome, and more effective. My daughter told me that I should try PHDS therapy. Since I started PHDS therapy, I am my old self again! My wife is delighted that I have regained my former "zip" that had been missing for so long."

—Mr. Robert from Missouri

"I am a husband, father, athlete, entrepreneur, volunteer, but during the past couple of years my physical and mental energy and sexual desire began to dramatically fall off. My wife was a patient of Dr. Tutera's and she was raving about her positive results with the PHDS therapy. I was too! She convinced me and the results have been beyond our expectations!

—Mr. Jim from California

Knowledge Is Power

Now that you have completed the reading of all the previous pages, you should know far more about how your body works, how to communicate better with your physician and ask for proper diagnostic tests and how to distinguish equivalent from bio-equivalent HRT options. You should also understand the powerful and dynamic benefits PHDS therapy can provide. equivalent hormones are the only choice if you want to reinvigorate your life without the nasty side effects of the more traditional HRT treatment options. Your body wants what it originally was designed to have. equivalent, natural, subcutaneous pellet therapy is the only HRT option that will reestablish a normal hormonal process in your body. The pellet hormone delivery system therapy will enable you to enjoy:

- A restored sexual drive
- Relief from hormone-related depression
- Consistency! No more roller-coaster effect compared to oral therapies and/or injections
- Elevated energy levels
- Greater capacity for getting in shape
- Increased mental clarity and focus
- Substantially diminished fears and frustrations concerning traditional HRT

The only form of hormone therapy that is truly effective with a few minor side-effects, is PHDS therapy. I am dedicated to making this form of therapy available to every woman and man for replacement of those precious hormones that benefit, protect, and energize our lives. Pellet hormone therapy has been utilized in the United States since 1939 but has never caught on because of the popularity of synthetic compounds and horse hormone. It's time for a change. If you are like most patients I see, you are probably anxious to find a physician who can help you with PHDS therapy. There is a growing list of physicians who are using PHDS therapy and who have also been trained by me in the full and complete processes of diagnosis and extensive monitoring of this type of therapy.

I have enjoyed sharing my insights and experience with you over the course of these pages. Whatever you do, please remember that a healthy, well-balanced and exciting life can once again be yours.

Nutritional Supplements

I know there are numerous authors touting their supplements, but nutritional supplements can be dangerous through overuse.

Pregnenalone and dehydroepiandrosterone (DHEA) carry definite risks and should only be used if nothing else is available, and only in

A healthy, well-balanced and exciting life can be yours once again.

strict moderation. Medline defines DHEA as an endogenous hormone (made in the human body) that is secreted by the adrenal gland. DHEA serves as precursor to male and female sex hormones (androgens and estrogens). DHEA levels in the body begin to decrease after age thirty and are reported to be low in some people with anorexia, end-stage kidney disease, type two diabetes (non-insulin dependent diabetes), AIDS, adrenal insufficiency, and in the critically ill. DHEA levels may also be depleted by a number of drugs, including insulin, corticosteroids, opiates, and danazol.

There is sufficient evidence supporting the use of DHEA in the treatment of adrenal insufficiency, depression, induction of labor, and systemic lupus erythematosus. No studies on the long-term effects of DHEA have been conducted. DHEA can cause higher than normal levels of androgens and estrogens in the body and, theoretically, may increase the risk of prostate, breast, ovarian, and other hormone-sensitive cancers. Therefore, it is not recommended for regular use without supervision by a licensed health professional.

With the scheme of how our bodies make estrogen and testosterone, you need to realize that all the other substances offered as supplements, often taken in combination, can cause physiologic harm to our bodies. Pregnenalone and DHEA both help the body make testosterone, but no study has been done to establish a safe amount of either compound. If you have a normal estrogen and testosterone level in the blood your body doesn't need DHEA or Pregnenalone. The following list of common nutritional supplements and the symptoms they may treat may help you to understand more about them. Always check with your physician before using any nutritional supplement to treat menopause symptoms.

Nutritional Supplement	Symptoms
Marine Photoplankton	Provides raw materials that promote the healthy functioning of cells, improves memory and mental functioning, and minimizes menopause symptoms such as mood swings and depression.
Flaxseed Oil	Depression and fatigue, may help to lower cholesterol and boost the immune system
Evening Primrose	Helps to alleviate common perimenopause symptoms such as irritation, water retention, cramping and headaches.
Coral Calcium	Provides an alkalizing effect on the body that may help to reduce acidity levels in the body, promoting calm and restoring balance.
Vitamin B6	Increases levels of sertonin and progesterone in the body, which helps reduce anxiety.
Go-ji (lyceum)	May help to restore kidney health and therefore promote hormonal balance.

Vitamin E	May help to alleviate a variety of menopause-related symptoms, and is therefore considered to be a mild form of hormone replacement therapy (HRT)
Vitamin C	May help to strengthen the immune system.
Zinc	May help to increase levels of progesterone and decrease levels of estrogen, boost the immune system; reduces the risk of osteoporosis.

Chapter 10

The First Day of the Rest of Your Life

"The best and safest thing is to keep a balance in your life and acknowledge the great powers around us and in us. If you can do that, and live that way, you are a really wise man."
—Euripides, 484 B.C.

Remember when your sex drive was healthy, you felt great, slept like a baby and had more energy than you knew what to do with? Back then, you didn't worry about things like osteoporosis, heart health or even cancer. Those were old folks' maladies.

But now that you are experiencing the life-altering symptoms of menopause or andropause, the outlook for aging gracefully looks a lot less hopeful, doesn't it? What wouldn't you give to have your happy, healthy, vivacious life back?

The plain truth is you <u>can</u> have it back with equivalent PHDS Therapy. Our equivalent hormone therapy was designed specifically to help you achieve the natural, healthy balance of estrogen and testosterone your body needs to maintain optimum well-being. PHDS therapy actually replenishes what is lost in the aging process, using the equivalent hormones your body used to create when you were healthy and in your prime.

Imagine feeling like you're thirty-something again! Within just a short time of beginning your PHDS Therapy, symptoms will start to disappear—the fatigue, the hot flashes, the foggy thinking and restless nights will all vanish. Instead, you'll feel like your sexy "young" self again.

Throughout this book, I have tried to establish that there are two critical factors in achieving good hormonal health and optimal well-being:

1. The use of natural equivalent hormones delivered by the pellet hormone delivery system (PHDS)
   a. A safe and effective alternative to synthetic or other hormone replacement therapies delivered in a worry-free, liver-safe, continuous, on-demand way.
   b. Confidence that you are receiving the right dosage of hormones for your body at all times.
   c. No other form of hormone delivery—whether micronized capsules, pills, creams, or patches can produce the consistent blood level of estrogen and testosterone that the PHDS can. This consistent level of hormone will give you the same sense of being and vitality you felt in your thirties.
   d. The longer you use the PHDS therapy, the more results you will see and feel.
   e. As your body returns to normalized function, you will sleep better, think more clearly, and enjoy an increase in your life.
   f. Without hot flashes or erectile dysfunction, you will feel like the new OLD you again.
2. Hormonal balance
   • Regain peace of mind.

The medical community has worked diligently over the last decades to be able to provide this modality of treatment, which is accessible to women of all lifestyles everywhere.

Are you a candidate for this life-enhancing affordable treatment?

- Do you want your vague feelings of depression to be gone?
- Do you want to face each day with renewed joy?
- Do you want to look in the mirror and see a beautiful smiling you?
- Do you want to walk into the future sure-footed and determined to reap all that the world offers?

Talk with your physician today and reap the many benefits of this kind of therapy, which is right within your reach.

To locate a SottoPelle® physician trained in the PHDS, visit the Web site at: www.sottopellesociety.com.

Frequently Asked Questions (FAQs)

1. What makes PHDS the preferred method of hormone replacement therapy?

PHDS Therapy delivers the right kind of hormone (biologically equivalent), in the right amounts (based on testing & proper analysis of the results), using the right delivery system (pellets).

- *Completely natural hormone replacement*
- *Decreased body fat and greater capacity to get in shape*
- *Relief from anxiety and depression*
- *Increased energy, focus, mental clarity and concentration—no more "foggy thinking"*
- *Increased sexual arousal and sex drive*
- *Increased bone density*

- *Works in partnership with your body twenty-four/seven*
- *No patches or creams*
- *Virtually no side effects and hassle-free*
- *Lasts up to six months*
- *This method of equivalent hormone replacement therapy has been documented and researched in medical journals since 1939*

2. Why are hormonal deficiencies so well corrected by the pellet hormone delivery system?

Normal levels of each hormone are achieved in the blood utilizing very low doses of estadiol (estrogen) and testosterone. In order for other hormone therapies (i.e., capsules, creams and sublingual tablets) to be effective, they often must be administered in high doses twice a day. Many women receive anywhere from one hundred fifty mg to three hundred mg a month in order to "feel better." With some of the tablets, there is the added problem of incorrect compounding, which causes them to dissolve improperly, thus rendering them useless.

Because the pellet hormone delivery system is not absorbed in your stomach, then processed by your liver, higher doses can be administered. Biologically equivalent estrogen and testosterone are delivered in the right amount at the right time without subjecting you to excess medicine.

The pellet hormone delivery system releases estrogen (estradiol) and testosterone directly into the blood stream, thereby bypassing the liver. This is the way the body has always received its hormones—in a steady amount that is secreted into the bloodstream from the ovaries or testicles. The body needs those levels of estrogen and testosterone in the bloodstream at all times in order to function optimally. When you receive hormone replacement therapy in the form of pills—whether synthetic or natural or equivalent —they must go through the stomach and liver. This process takes longer to get estrogen and testosterone into your system; it also means that the bloodstream must receive much larger doses in order for there to be any hormone available to help the body at the end of its journey. It also makes it unlikely that the natural two to one ratio it needs for optimal health will occur. The only hormone replacement therapy to deliver estrogen and testosterone in this manner for a prolonged period of time (four to six months) is the PHDS equivalent therapy.

The PHDS therapy is the only form of hormone replacement therapy that can release more hormones when the body demands it. Pills, creams, and even micronized capsules limit what your body can receive in a specific time period. Once you have used up your dose, that's it. You must either take another capsule, or use more cream. That means you experience peaks and valleys in your hormone levels. Instead of the steady stream of hormone your body once produced it now gets first a lot, then a little, then none.

If you are on the patch or receive shots, these methods are also incapable of responding to an immediate hormone demand. Bottom line—when the body says it needs more it doesn't automatically get it. The great thing about the pellet hormone delivery system is that it does respond when your body says, I need more hormone. When a message goes out from the brain that says I'm stressed or I need to repair some muscles or I need to build some bone, the pellets respond immediately releasing more estrogen or testosterone. The body gets what it asks for.

PHDS therapy is made of pure crystallized, biologically equivalent estradiol (estrogen) and testosterone. The PHDS pellets are specially formulated for the clinic by a compounding pharmacy, using the purest ingredients and manufactured to the highest standards. Both the estradiol (estrogen) and the testosterone are derived from soy and other natural plant-based ingredients. They possess the exact hormonal structure of the human hormone.

3. How can I tell if I need hormone replacement therapy?

Simply put, the only way to tell you are hormone deficient is through testing and proper analysis of the results. Hormone balance cannot be accomplished with guesswork or based on insufficient information. It is critical to your diagnosis that your doctor order the correct lab work and understand what the results indicate—which is too often not the case.

PHDS Therapy is based on a thorough understanding of how the human endocrine system works and what it needs to maintain balance. Once your hormone levels are accurately measured and analyzed, you will receive the proper dose of equivalent hormone through the PHDS to fulfill your body's requirements. Your hormone levels will thereafter be tested periodically in order to assess the ongoing success of your hormone replacement therapy. There is no guesswork or "one size fits all" with PHDS therapy.

4. How is this treatment given?

The procedure is simple. Using a local anesthetic, the estrogen and testosterone pellets are individually placed painlessly under the skin in the hip or buttock area. From start to finish, it takes less than five minutes.

5. Will I need to use this treatment for the rest of my life?

There is no reason that you cannot use this therapy forever. I have a large number of patients who have used pellet therapy between ten and twenty-five years. They are physically well while acting and looking younger than their age.

6. Are there any long-term problems associated with this therapy?

I have not seen any long-term problems. In fact, would they still be using pellets since 1939 if there are long-term problems?

7. What is the youngest age that the pellet hormone delivery system can be used?

I have used testosterone pellets in a seventeen-year-old young man who had low testosterone levels. The youngest woman was eighteen years of age and treated for menstrual migraine headaches successfully using pellet therapy.

8. Can you explain how this type of therapy may help with PMS?

Pellets can be used to stabilize estrogen levels by giving steady estrogen levels, thereby stopping the wide swings of estrogen which produces PMS.

9. Are there any dietary restrictions while using the pellet hormone delivery system?

No, there are not any dietary restrictions while using pellets. As a matter of fact, the testosterone pellets will help you feel more energized, thus giving you the energy to exercise!

10. Can you use this therapy while taking thyroid hormones and or heart or blood pressure medicines?

Since the hormones are not processed in the liver, medicines will not be affected by pellet use. I myself have been on pellets for over seven years and take thyroid hormone. I also have an irregular heart rhythm which requires my using heart medication and blood thinner. I have had no problems with the pellets affecting my medications.

11. Why don't you use dehydroepiandrosterone (DHEA)?

DHEA is a precursor for testosterone, and if your testosterone is normal you don't make as much DHEA. Unfortunately DHEA can be transformed into Estrone and Dihydrotestosterone (DHT) which can cause breast and prostate problems.

12. Why don't you use HGH?

HGH is a hormone that is being given to patients to do the things that testosterone does in the human body. Unlike testosterone pellets, HGH shots cause insulin resistance which raises the chance of developing high blood pressure, heart attack, stroke, and diabetes. It also will cause tumors to grow in the breast, prostate, brain, etc. It also can affect thyroid function causing hypothyroidism. Finally, it increases the production of T.N.F. (tumor necroisis factor) that accelerates the spread of all types of cancer cells (metastasis). HGH is a very dangerous hormone and should not be used in human beings except for its approved user: 1) Dwarfism and 2) Treatment after Pituitary Tumor Removal.

13. What possible side effects are there?

The side effects in both men and women are rare. In women transient breast tenderness lasting 7-10 days may occur with the first insertion, but rarely with repeat treatments. Acne and hair loss are rare occurrences from testosterone therapy. The growth of facial hair is also rare, and occurs no more frequently than what happens in post menopausal women on no hormones. In men, the side effects are rare but may include decreased sperm count, decreased testicular mass, and possible prostate enlargement.

14. How many patients have you treated with pellet hormones?

I have patients who come to see me from around the world. I have treated more than 15,000 patients who state their lives have been changed in a positive way. Please keep in mind that individual results may vary.

References

1. Israni RK. Hormone Therapy in Menopause Called Safer if Early. *Med Page Today*. View at www.medpagetoday.com/OBGYN/HRT/tb/5384.
2. Greenblatt RB, Bryner JR. Estradiol Pellet Implantation in the Management of Menopause. *The Journal of Reproductive Medicine*.1977;18:307-316.
3. Bishop PM. A clinical experiment in estrin therapy. Br Med. 1938;1:939.
4. Gambrell RD, Natrajan PK. Moderate dosage estrogen-androgen therapy improves continuation rates in postmenopausal women: impact of the WHI reports.*CLIMACTERIC*.2006;9;224-233.
5. Gambrell RD. Management of hormone replacement side effects. *Menopause*.1994;1:67-72.

6. Soares CN. Menopause and Mood Disturbance. Psychiatric Times.2005;1. View at www.psychiatrictimes.com/showArticle.jhtml?articleID=60400124.

7. Wise PM, Krajnak KM, Kashon ML. Menopause: the aging of multiple pacemakers. *Science*.1996;273:67-70.

8. AACE menopause Guidelines Revision Task Force. American Association of Clinical Endocrinologists Medical Guidelines for Clinical Practice for the Diagnosis and Treatment of Menopause. *Endocr Pract.* 2006;12:315-337.

9. Heard MJ. The Latest Facts About Premature Ovarian Failure. 2003. View at www.drdonnica.com/guests/oooo6208.htm.

10. Smith NJ, Studd JW. Recent advances in hormone replacement therapy. *British Journal of Hospital Medicine.* 1993;11:799-808.

11. Dubey RK, Jackson EK. Estrogen-induced cardiorenal protection: potential cellular, biochemical, and molecular mechanisms. *Am J Physiol Renal Physiol.* 2001;280:F365-F388.

12. Savvas M, Studd JW, Norman S, et al. Increase in bone mass after one year of percutaneous oestradiol and testosterone implants in post-menopausal women who have previously received long-term oral oestrogens. *British Journal of Obstetrics and Gynecology.* 1992;99:757-760.

13. Anawalt BD, Merriam GR. Neuroendocrine again in men. Andropause and somatopause. *Endocrinol Metab Clin North Am.* 2001;30:647-669.

14. Turek PJ. Androgens and the Aging Male. 2005. View at: http://urology.ucsf.edu/patient guides/pdf/maleInf/Androgens.pdf..

15. Bachmann G, Bancroft J, Braunstein G, et al. Female androgen insufficiency: the Princeton consensus statement on definition, classification, and assessment. *Fertility and Sterility.*2002;4:660-665.

16. Medscape. Conclusion: Empiric vs Low-Dose Adjustive Hormone Replacement Therapy. 2001. View at

http://www.medscape.com/viewarticle/412853_6.

17. Studd TM. Oestorgen/testosterone implant therapy. *Oestrogens and the Menopause*.1978.

18. Smith RN, Studd JW. *British Journal of Hospital Medicine*. 1993.

19. Elkik F, Gompel A. MTP Press. 103-125.

20. Handelsman DJ. *Pharmacology, Biology, and Clinical Applications of Androgen*. 1994.

21. Magos A, Zilkha KJ, Studd JW. Treatment of menstrual migraine by oestradiol implants. Journal of Neurology, Neurosurgery, and Psychiatry. 1983;46:1044-1046.

22. Studd J, Savvas M, Waston N, et al. The relationship between plasma estradiol and the increase in bone density in post menopausal women after treatment with subcutaneous hormone implants. *Am J Obstet Gynecol*. 1990;163:1474-1479.

23. Natrajan PK, Gambrell RD. Estrogen replacement therapy in patients with early breast cancer. *American Journal of Obstetrics and Gynbecology*. 2002;189.

24. Bush NJ. Advances in hormonal therapy for breast cancer. *Semin Oncol Nurs*. 2007;23:46-54.

25. Smith RN, Studd JW. Recent advances in hormone replacement therapy. *Br J Hosp Med*. 1993;49:799-808.

26. Westhoff C, Britton J, Gammon M, et al. Oral contraceptive and benign ovarian tumors.*Am J Epidemiol*. 2000;152:242-246.

27. Tan RS. The Andropause Mystery:Unraveling the Truths About Male Menopause. Publisher *AMRED*.2001.

28. Tan RS, Pu SJ. Is it andropause? Recognizing androgen deficiency in aging men. *Postgrad Med*. 2004;115:62-22.

29. Lindsey R, Hart D, Aitken J, et al. Long-term prevention of post-menopausal osteoporosis by oestrogen. Evidence for an increased bone mass after delayed onset of oestrogen treatment. *Lancet*. 1976;1:1038-1041.

30. Dobs A. Role of testosterone in maintaining lean body mass and bone density in HIV-infected patients. *Int J Impot Res*.

2003;4:521-525.

31   Bouic P. *The Immune System Cure*.

32   Nightingale SL. From the Food and Drug Administration. *JAMA*.1997;278:1394.

33.   Bartalena, L. Effects of thyroxine excess on peripheral organs. *Acta Med Austriaca*, 21 (2): 60-65, 1994.

34.   Braverman, Lewis E., Robert D. Utiger. *Werner and Ingbar's The Thyroid: A Fundamental and Clinical Text*. 7th Edition. Lippincot-Raven. 1996.

35.   L.J. DeGroot, P.R. Larsen, S. Refetoff, and J.B. Stanbury: *The Thyroid and Its Diseases*, 5th edition. New York, John Wiley & Sons, Inc. 1984, pp.577-578.

36.   Fallon, M. D. Exogenous hyperthyroidism with osteoporosis. Arch. Intern. Med., 143: 442-444, 1983.

37.   Hamburger, J. I.: Strategies for cost effective thyroid function testing with modern methods. Diagnostic Methods in Clinical Throidology. 1989, pp. 63-109

38.   Korsic, M. Bone mineral density in patients on long term therapy with Levothyroxine. *Lijec Vjesn*, 120 (5): 103-05, 1988.

39.   Lowe, J.C.: *The Metabolic Treatment of Fibromyalgia*. Boulder, 2000.

40.   Paul, T. L. Long term L-thyroxine therapy is associated with decreased hip-bone density in premenopausal women. JAMA, 259: 3137-3141. 1988.

41.   Toft, A. D.: Thyroxine replacement treatment: clinical judgment or biochemical control? Br. Med. J., 291: 233, 1985.

42.   Shapiro, L. E.: Minimal cardiac effects in asymptomatic athyreotic patients chronically treated with thyrotropin-suppressive doses of l-thyroxine. J. Clin. Endocrinol. Metab., 82 (8):2592-2595, 1997.

43.   Skinner, G. R. B.: Thyroxine should be tried in clinically hypothyroid but biochemically euthyroid patients (letter). Brit. Med. J., 314:1764, 1997.

44. Tjørve, E. Tjørve, K.M., Olsen, J.O., et al.: On commonness and rarity of thyroid hormone resistance: A discussion based on mechanisms of reduced sensitivity in peripheral tissues. *Medical Hypotheses*, Mar 23, 2007. Lillehammer University College, 2626 Lillehammer, Norway.

45. Vanderpump MPJ, Tunbridge WMG, French JM, Appleton D, Bates M, Clark F, et al. The incidence of thyroid disorders in the community: a twenty-year follow-up of the Whickham survey. *Clin Endocrinol* 1995; 43: 55-68

46. Dowling D. The Hormone Connection to Women's Health. SelfGrowth.com. Viewed at http://www.selfgrowth.com/articles/Dowling1.html, September 2007.

47. Willhite L. Urogenital Atrophy: Prevention and Treatment. *Pharmacotherapy.*2001.21;464-480.

48. Concensus Conference. Osteoporosis. *JAMA.*1984;252:799-802.

49. Burch J, Byrd B, Vaughn W. Results of estrogen treatment in one thousand hysterectomized women for 14,318 years. In: van Keep PA, Greenblatt R, Albeaus-Fernet M, eds. Consensus on menopause research. Lancaster, Eng.:MTP Press, 1976:164-169.

50. *Am J Ophthalmol.* 2002;134:842-848.

51. Dellolacono T. Nutrition and Menopause. MenopauseRX. Viewed at www.menopauserx.com/health_center/well_nutrition.htm.

Additional Reading

Androgen Therapy. National Women's Health Resource Center. View at www.healthywomen.org.

Ansbacher R. Estrogen and estrogen-Like Substances. *Postgraduate Obstetrics & Gynecology.* 1998;12:1-5.

Bachmann GA. The hypoandrogenic woman: pathophysiologic overview. *Fertility and Sterility.* 2002;4:S72-S76.

Burger HG, Hailes J, Menelalus M, et al. The management of persistent menopausal symptoms with oestradiol-testosterone implants: clinical, lipid and hormonal results. *Maturitas.* 1984;6:351-358.

Burger H. Hormone replacement therapy in the post-Women's Health Initiative era. Report of a meeting held in Funchal, Madeira, February 24-25, 2003. *Climacteric*.2003;1:11-36.

Cameron D, Braunstein G. Androgen replacement therapy in women. *Fertility and Sterility*. 2004;2:273-288.

Cardozo L, Gibb D, Tuck S, et al. The effects of subcutaneous hormone implants during the climacteric. *Maturitas*. 1984;5:177-184.

Collins W, Studd J. Hormonal Profiles in Postmenopausal Women After Therapy with Subcutaneous Implants. *British Journal of Obstetrics and Gynecology*.1981. 8:426-433.

Cravioto M, Larrea F, Delgado N, et al. Pharmacokinetics and pharmacodynamics of 25-mg estradiol implants in postmenopausal Mexican women. *Menopause*. 2001;3:353-360.

Davis S, McCloud P, Strauss B, Burger H. Testosterone enhances estradiol's effects on postmenopausal bone density and sexuality. *Maturitas*. 1995;21:227-236.

Davis S. Rationale for Treating Hypoandrogenism in Women. Contemporary Endocrinology: Androgens in Health and Disease.1987;8:1-28. Published by Humana Press Inc. Totowa, NJ.

Davis S, Walker K, Strauss B. Effects of estradiol with and without testosterone on body composition and relationships with lipids in postmenopausal women. *Menopause*. 2000;6:395-401.

Davis S. When to suspect androgen deficiency other than at menopause. *Fertility and Sterility*. 2002;4:S68-S71.

Farish F, Fletcher C, Hart D, et al. The effects of hormone implants on serum lipoproteins and steroid hormones in bilaterally oophorectomised women. *Acta Endocrinologica.* 1984;106:116-120.

Greenblatt R, Asch R, Mahesh V, Dryner J. Implantation of pure crystalline pellets of estradiol for conception contron. *Am J Obstet Gynecol.* 1977;127:520-524.

Harman SM. Estrogen replacement in menopausal women: recent and current prospective studies, the WHI and the KEEPS. *Gend Med.* 2006;3:254-269.

Leonetti H, Longo S, Anasti J. Transdermal Progesterone Cream for Vasomotor Symptoms and Postmenopausal Bone Loss. *Obstetrics and Gynecology.* 1999;94:225-228.

Lindsay R. Letter: Estrogen and bone loss. *Arch Intern Med.* 1976;136:1068.

Lobo R, March C, Goebelsmann U, et al. Effect upon serum estrone, estradiol, luteinizing hormone, follicle-stimulating hormone, corticosteroid binding globulin-binding capacity, testosterone-estradiol binding globulin-binging capacity, lipids, and hot flushes. *Am J Obstet Gynecol.* 1980;138:714-719.

Moffat S, Zonderman A, Metter E, et al. Free testosterone and risk for Alzheimer's disease in older men. *Neurology.* 2004;62:188-193.

Morley JE. Andropause, testosterone therapy , and quality of life in aging men. *Cleveland Clinic Journal of Medicine.* 2000;67:880-992.

Mrotek J. The Endocrine System. 2003; 4th Edition. The Endocrine Society, Chevy Chase, Maryland

Natrajan P, Soumakis K, Gambrell D. Estrogen replacement therapy in women with previous breast cancer. *Am J Obstet Gynecol.* 1999;181:288-295.

Notelovitz M, Johnston M, Smith S, Kitchens C. Metabolic and Hormonal Effects of 25-mg and 50-mg 17â-Estradiol Implants in Surgically Menopausal Women. *Obstet Gynecol.* 1897;70:749-754.

Paganini-Hill A. Alzheimer's Disease and Estrogen Replacement Therapy. *Postgraduate Obstetrics & Gynecology.* 1998;24:1-6.

Pirwany I, Sattar N, Greer I, et al. Supraphysiological concentrations of estradiol in menopausal women given repeated implant therapy do not adversely affect lipid profiles. *Human Reproduction.* 2002;3:825-829.

Shifren J, Desindes S, McIlwain M, et al. A randomized, open-label, crossover study comparing the effects of oral versus transdermal estrogen therapy on serum androgens, thyroid hormones, and adrenal hormones in naturally menopausal women. *Menopause.* 2007;15:

Singh M. Progestins and neuroprotection: are all progestins created equal? *Minerva Endocrinol.* 2007;32:95-102.

Ribot C, Tremollieres F. [Hormone replacement therapy in postmenopausal women: all the treatments are not the same.] *Gynecol Obstet Fertil.* 2007;3.

Savvas M, Studd J, Dooley M, Montgomery J. Comparison of oral and implanted oestrogens for their effects in preventing postmenopausal osteoporosis. *BMJ.* 1988;331-333.

Stanczyk F, Shoupe D, Nunez V, et al. A randomized comparison of nonoral estradiol delivery in postmenopausal women. *Am J Obstet Gynecol.* 1988;159:1540-1546.

Tan R, Phhilip P. Perceptions of and risk factors for andropause. *Archives of Andrology.* 1999;43:227-233.

Thorneycroft IH. The role of estrogen replacement therapy in the prevention of osteoporosis. *Am J Obstet Gynecol.* 1989;160:1306-1310.

Thyroid Web Resource:

Nature-Throid™: http://www.rlclabs.com

After Statement

If you are a woman or a man seeking an end to your fears about and frustrations with hormone replacement therapy, I trust that this book will assist you in your search for a physician who will meet your needs. If you are a physician who is tired of going through the routine without fulfilling results, I invite you to read this book carefully and contact me for any additional data or research.

Gino Tutera, MD, FACOG
www.sottopelletherapy.com

About the Author

GINO TUTERA, MD, FACOG

Gino Tutera, MD has more than thirty years of experience as a specialist in treating PMS, menopause, and hormonal imbalance. He has pioneered an unbelievable medical breakthrough with the pellet hormone delivery system for hormonal therapy, which is changing the lives of thousands of men and women around the Country.

Dr. Tutera has completed ten years of documented research on the reduction of breast and ovarian cancer with pellet hormone delivery system therapy.

Dr. Tutera was born in Rome, Italy and grew up in Kansas City, Missouri. He received his medical training at the University of Missouri in Columbia, Missouri. He then became Chief Resident at St. Luke's Hospital in Kansas City, Missouri in 1974.

At the forefront of his peers, Dr. Tutera opened his first clinic devoted to hormonal replacement and PMS in 1982. His corporate office is located in

Scottsdale, Arizona, with his newest offices in Gilbert and Paradise Valley, Arizona. He still retains his original PHDS office in Rancho Mirage, California. Dr. Tutera is committed to elevating PHDS therapy to a level where it is available for every woman and man in America who wants and needs it.

"It's the only hormone replacement therapy that makes sense for normal breast health."
—Nedra Harrison, MD, breast cancer surgeon

"I have been using the pellet hormone delivery system therapy since 2000. I have never felt so good—my anxieties have disappeared, I have more energy, my hair and skin are better. I feel happy and calm. Thank goodness for Dr. Gino Tutera."
—Keely Smith, celebrity and singer

Currently, Medical Director of SottoPelle®—Center for Hormonal Balance & Well-Being, with locations throughout Arizona, with the corporate office located in Scottsdale, Arizona and Rancho Mirage, California.

Licensure

State of Missouri, 1971
State of California, 1993
State of Arizona, 2000
Medical Director of OB/GYN at Baptist
Medical Center, Kansas City, MO, 1981-1984
Medical Director of Kansas City PMS Clinic, 1982-1992
Medical Director, Women's Center at Baptist
Medical Center, Kansas City, MO, 1982—Created center dealing
    with women's health issues including education and reference
    library
Clinical Instructor for Obstetrics & Gynecology

Goppert Family Practice Residency, 1984-1987

Medical Director of the Hanson Birthing Center, Obstetrical Unit at Eisenhower Medical Center, Rancho Mirage, California 1992-1995

Chairman, Section of OB/GYN at Eisenhower Medical Center Rancho Mirage, California 1996-1998

Vice Chairman, Department of Obstetrics & Gynecology, Baptist Medical Center, Kansas City, Missouri, 1989-1991

Diplomat of American Board of Obstetrics & Gynecology, 1977-Present

Fellow American College of Obstetrics & Gynecology, 1977-Present

Medical Society Memberships

Diplomat American Board of Obstetrics & Gynecology
Fellow American College of Obstetrics & Gynecology
American Medical Association
California Medical Association
Missouri Medical Association
American Association of Gynecologic
Laparoscopists
American Society of Colposcopy and
Cervical Pathology
Author, *You Don't Have to Live With It*

Glossary

A

Achilles—Tendon at back of ankle

Amniotic Fluid—Fluid surrounding the unborn fetus during pregnancy

Anabolic Steroids—Hormones related to testosterone

Androgens—Hormones that have male hormone effects in the human body (i.e., DHEA, Testosterone, etc.)

Andropause—Male menopause

Antiatherogenic—Protection against the formation of plaques

Adrenocorticotropic hormone (ACTH) —A hormone from a gland in the brain called the pituitary. It regulates the adrenal glands in the body

Addison's Disease—A disease of the adrenal glands. This life threatening disease results from the adrenal glands being unable to produce cortisol, the body's cortisone

Alzheimer's Disease—A form of dementia

Androgen—Any natural or synthetic compound, usually a synthetic hormone, that stimulates or controls the development of masculine traits in vertebrates

Andrology—Medical specialty that deals with the problems of the male reproductive system

Andropause—"Male Menopause." The male body is no longer able to produce enough testosterone

Androstenedione—(An-dro-steen-dye-own) a hormone that has weaker male effects than testosterone. Often seen as a supplement called "Andro," actually a hormone the body makes which is then transformed into testosterone and even estrogen

Antidiuretic hormone (ADH) —A small peptide molecule released by the pituitary gland

Aromatase—An enzyme in the human body that causes testosterone (a male hormone) to be changed to estrogen (female hormone) and vice versa.

Arrhythmia—Irregular heart rate pattern

Attention Deficit Disorder (ADD)—Most commonly diagnosed behavioral disorder

Atrophy—Loss of tissue thickness

Augment—To enlarge or to intensify an effect

Autoimmune—A condition that occurs when the immune system mistakenly attacks and destroys itself

B

Basal Body Temperature (BBT)—Body temperature measured immediately after awakening or before any physical activity

Bio-Available—The degree to which a drug is absorbed or becomes available

Bio-Equivalent—a term meaning a substance has effects similar to the biologic substance it's replacing, but does not have the exact chemical structure

Equivalent—a substance is equivalent to the substance it is replacing in both effect and chemical structure.

Biologically Equivalent—Equivalent to the human body

C

Cardiovascular—The circulatory system

Cerebral—Using the intellect rather than intuition

Chemical Messengers—Neurotransmitters transmitting impulses from one nerve cell to another

Cholesterol—a fat in the blood
HDL—the good cholesterol
LDL & VLDL—bad cholesterol

Chromosomal—Genetic conditions

Chronic Fatigue Syndrome (CFS)—A disorder causing extreme fatigue

Compounding pharmacy—A pharmacy that creates custom formulations of drugs according to a physician's orders

Conjugated Hormones—Synthetic hormones

Coronary Artery Disease (CAD) —A narrowing of the small blood vessels that supply blood and oxygen to the heart

Cortex—The outer shell of a body organ or gland

Cushing's Syndrome—A disease of the adrenal glands that causes the glands to over produce cortisol, causing high blood pressure, marked weight gain, muscle wasting,
fluid retention, and loss of bone density

D
Depression—A state of intense sadness

Diabetes—A disease caused by the pancreas not being able to produce enough insulin hormone so that the body can use sugars properly

Dehydroepiandrosterone (DHEA)—A weak male hormone produced by the body which is then changed into testosterone, the precursor to testosterone

Diagnosis—The act or process of identifying or determining the nature and cause of a disease or injury through evaluation of patient history, examination, and review of laboratory data

Duct—An often enclosed passage or channel for conveying a substance, especially a liquid or gas; a tubular bodily canal or passage, especially one for carrying a glandular secretion

Dysfunction—Abnormal or impaired functioning, especially of a bodily system or social group

E
Endocrine Glands—Any of various ductless glands such as the thyroid, adrenal, or pituitary, having hormonal secretions that pass directly into the bloodstream

Endocrine System—The body has a group of glands that secrete their hormones directly into the bloodstream and are called the endocrine system i.e.: the thyroid, pituitary, etc.

Endocrinology—The study of the endocrine glands and their function

Enzyme—A protein in the body that is used to start, speed up, or eliminate a particular chemical reaction in the body

Epinephrine—The other name for the body's "Adrenaline"

Equilin—The primary estrogen hormone in horses; the primary hormone in the drugs: Premarin™, Prempro™, and Premphase™

Erectile Dysfunction—The inability to achieve penile erection or to maintain an erection until ejaculation

Estradiol—The primary female hormone of the human body; the work-horse estrogen for human females

Estrogen—Female hormones

Estrogen deficiency—A lacking in one of the natural substances formed by the ovary, placenta, or testis

Estrone—One of the human female hormones, a very strong breast stimulator

Estriol—A very weak estrogen make from estrone

F

Feedback Mechanism—the system in the human body which regulates the creation and release of hormones from the endocrine glands

Fibromyalgia—A syndrome characterized by chronic pain in the muscles of soft tissues surrounding joints, fatigue, and tenderness at specific sites in the body

First Pass—First Pass Metabolism is the process in which the liver processes medicines in the liver cells

Follicle Stimulating Hormone (FSH)—The hormone made by the pituitary that regulates the female ovary and male testicle. It regulates the hormone production of these organs

Follicle Cells—Cells in the ovaries that produce estrogen

Follicular cells—Cells in the thyroid gland that produce thyroid hormone

G

Gastroesophageal Reflux Disease—A disease of the stomach and/or the esophagus

Genetic—Relating to genes; influenced by the origin or development of something

Geriatrician—A physician who deals with the diagnosis and treatment of diseases and problems specific to old age

Greenblatt, Robert, MD—one of the first physicians in America to use hormone pellets; first published his research in 1949

Growth Hormone (GH)—Somatotropin, a polypeptide hormone secreted by somatotrophs that promotes growth of the body

H

Homeostasis—The ability of tendency of an organism or a cell to maintain internal equilibrium by adjusting its physiological processes

Hormone—A substance, usually a peptide or steroid, produced by one tissue and conveyed by the bloodstream to another to effect physiological activity, such as growth or metabolism

Hormone Replacement Therapy (HRT)—The therapeutic administration of estrogen and perhaps other hormones to postmenopausal women to reduce the occurrence of hot flashes and to prevent osteoporosis and coronary disease

Hyperlipidemia—High cholesterol

Hyperthyroidism—The state of an overactive thyroid

Hypothyroidism—The state of an underactive thyroid

I

Insulin—the hormone produced by the pancreas (an endocrine gland) that regulates the body's blood sugar. A deficiency of insulin causes the disease diabetes

Insulin Resistance—A state of diminished effectiveness of insulin in lowering the levels of blood sugar, usually resulting from insulin binding by antibodies and associated with such conditions as obesity, ketoacidosis, and infection

Irritable Bowel Syndrome—Abnormally sensitive to stimulus

Islets of Langerhans—The cells in the pancreas that produce insulin

L

Lutenizing Hormone (LH)—The pituitary hormone that controls ovulation and progesterone hormone production in a woman, and testosterone in a man

M

Medulla—A term that refers to the middle of an organ or gland

Menopause—The time of life when a woman stops ovulating and stops producing enough estrogen, the female hormone

Menstrual Migraine—A severe headache that comes only around the time of a woman's menstrual period; probably caused by low estrogen levels

Metabolic—Relating to or resulting from metabolism

Metabolic Syndrome—Any insufficiency that affects the normal function of the metabolic system

Metabolism—The complex of physical and chemical processes occurring within a living cell or organism that are necessary for the maintenance of life

Musculoskeletal System—Relating to or involving the muscles and the skeleton

N

National Institutes of Health (NIH) —An agency of the United States Department of Health and Human Services dedicated to medical research

Neurotransmitter—Any of the various chemical substances, such as acetylcholine, that transmits nerve impulses across a synapse

Norepinephrine—the other adrenaline the adrenal glands produce

Nutrition—The process by which a living organism assimilates food and uses it for growth, liberation of energy, and replacement of tissues

O

OB/GYN (Obstetrics and Gynecology)—The medical field dedicated to the care of women during and after pregnancy

Osteopenia—Decreased bone density sufficient enough to increase the fracture risk in human bones

Osteoporosis—A disease in which the bones become extremely porous, are subject to fractures, and heal slowly, occurring especially in women following menopause and often leading to curvature of the spine from vertebral collapse

Ovary—The female reproductive endocrine organ. The ovaries are positioned one on each side of the uterus

Ovulation—The process of expelling the female egg from the ovary

Ovarian Cancer—Cancer of the ovaries

Oxytocin—A short polypeptide hormone that is released from the posterior lobe of the pituitary gland, and stimulates the contraction of smooth muscle of the uterus during labor, and facilitates release of milk from the breast during nursing

P

Pancreas—The endocrine organ that is located in the belly that produces digestive enzymes, and the hormone insulin

Pathophysiology—The functional changes associated with or resulting from disease or injury

Pellet Hormone Delivery System (PHDS)—A subcutaneous means for delivering hormones throughout the body in a safe, continuous flow avoiding the liver

Pharmaceutical Hormones—Synthetic hormones

Physiologic—Being in accord with or characteristic of the normal functioning of a living organism

Post Partum Depression (PPD)—Severe sadness occurring in the period shortly after childbirth

Premature Ovary Failure (POF)—The occurrence of ovary failure before menopause when the ovaries cease to produce estrogen

Pregnenalone—A hormone made from progesterone which the body creates on the way to making estrogen and testosterone

Progesterone—The hormone produced from the ovary after the egg has been expelled. Usually only produced in significant amounts for ten to twelve days of each menstrual cycle. High levels are only seen in pregnancy

Prolactin (PRL)—The hormone produced by the back portion of the pituitary gland (posterior pituitary) which causes milk production and milk let down from the female breast

Prolapse—A term used to indicate a loss of support for the uterus, (i.e.: uterine prolapse) which caused the uterus to drop lower into the vagina

Psychological—Of or relating to, or arising from the mind or emotions

Pulmonary Embolus—A usually fatal condition caused by a blood clot being released (thrown) to the lung, commonly from the leg veins or pelvic veins

R

Rectal Incontinence—The loss of control of the anal sphincter muscle which causes fecal material to exit

Reproduction—The sexual or asexual process by which organisms generate others of the same kind

"Roller-coaster Effect"—The up and down of hormone levels produced by pills, patches, creams and shots; does not occur with PHDS

S

Salivary Glands—Glands in the mouth that produce saliva (spit) and deliver it through a tiny tube called a duct

Serotonin—An organic compound formed from tryptophan and found in animals and human tissue, especially the brain, blood serum, and gastric mucous membranes, and active in vasoconstriction, stimulation of the smooth muscles, transmission of impulses between nerve cells, and regulation of cyclic body processes

Sex Hormone Binding Globulin (SHBG)—A steroid hormone, such as estrogen and androgen, affecting the growth or function of the reproductive organs and the development of secondary sex characteristics; a protein which can attach itself to estrogen or testosterone and make them unavailable for the body to absorb from the blood

Sheehan's Syndrome—Results from a partial or complete loss of blood supply to the pituitary gland. This results in partial or complete loss of the pituitary's ability to produce its hormones, and can lead to the loss of thyroid hormone, estrogen hormone production, testosterone production, and adrenal gland function which could result in serious illness or death if not properly treated

Subcutaneous—"Under the skin"; the fatty layer that lies just under the skin

Surgical Menopause—Menopause caused to happen instantly by the removal of the ovaries at any age; estrogen ceases to secrete

Synthetic hormone—Any hormone not of natural origin

T

Testicle—The male sex gland; it produces sperm and testosterone hormones

Testosterone—The male hormone; an androgen

Thyroid Gland—A two-lobed endocrine gland located in front of and on either side of the trachea and producing various hormones, such as calcitonin

Thyroid Stimulating Hormone (TSH)—The hormone produced by the pituitary gland that controls the creation and release of the two thyroid hormones

Triodothyronine (T3)—One of two thyroid hormones

Thyroxine (T4)—One of two thyroid hormones

U

Urinary Incontinence—The inability to control the loss of urine from the bladder

V

Vaginal Atrophy—The loss of the normal lining and the thickness of the vagina, which makes a woman feel dry and causes discomfort during sexual intercourse

W

Women's Health Initiative (WHI)—A major fifteen-year research program established in 1991 to address the most common causes of

death, disability and poor quality of life in postmenopausal women—
cardiovascular disease, cancer, and osteoporosis